# Leukaemia - Recent Advances in Diagnosis and Therapeutic Modalities

*Edited by Marwa Zakaria, Samar Elbahy, Al Zahraa Allam and Hanan Yousif Al-Abboh*

Published in London, United Kingdom

Leukaemia - Recent Advances in Diagnosis and Therapeutic Modalities
http://dx.doi.org/10.5772/intechopen.1008633
Edited by Marwa Zakaria, Samar Elbahy, Al Zahraa Allam and Hanan Yousif Al-Abboh

Contributors
Alan Chew-Bonilla, Dao-Hai Cheng, Dmytro Gur`yanov, Emiliano Fulda Graue, Federico Graue Wiechers, Gennadii Telegeev, Ibrahim O. Ahmed, Irene Gartovska, Jorge Morales-Navarro, Jun Du, Kaladada I. Korubo, Lyudmyla P. Shvachko, Maria Renee Jimenez-Sotomayor, Michael Zavelevich, Muheez A. Durosinmi, Mykhailo Dybkov, Rahman A. Bolarinwa, Shivani Golem, Svitlana Antonenko, Wen-Ling Chen, Zou-Fang Huang



First published in London, United Kingdom, 2026 by IntechOpen
IntechOpen is the global imprint of INTECHOPEN LIMITED, registered in England and Wales, registration number: 11086078, 167-169 Great Portland Street, London, W1W 5PF, United Kingdom

For EU product safety concerns: IN TECH d.o.o., Prolaz Marije Krucifikse Kozulić 3, 51000 Rijeka, Croatia, info@intechopen.com or visit our website at intechopen.com.

British Library Cataloguing-in-Publication Data
A catalogue record for this book is available from the British Library

Leukaemia - Recent Advances in Diagnosis and Therapeutic Modalities
Edited by Marwa Zakaria, Samar Elbahy, Al Zahraa Allam and Hanan Yousif Al-Abboh
p. cm.

This title is part of the Oncology Book Series, Volume 15
Topic: Hemato-oncology
Series Editor: Thomas J. FitzGerald
Topic Editor: Seema Naik

Print ISBN 978-1-80631-013-5
Online ISBN 978-1-80631-012-8
eBook (PDF) ISBN 978-1-80631-014-2
ISSN 3049-8864

# IntechOpen Book Series
# Oncology
## Volume 15

## Aims and Scope of the Series

The field of oncology has undergone extraordinary change and progress over the past several decades. Today, information is evolving at a rapid rate, with standards of management far different than standards of care applied during the training of most practicing oncologists. Oncology practitioners in all disciplines must remain current to optimize patient care. Basic and translational science remain critical in developing process improvements for patient care. The closer we understand the mechanism, the more we can improve targeted therapies and apply them to patient care. The pace of information is moving faster than at any previous time in history, and all oncology disciplines must remain current to provide excellent service to patients. The modern oncologist must be fluent in using big data and the volume of information generated in clinical trials. As we move closer to personalized patient care based on genomics and molecular biomarkers, the modern oncologist has to be nimble in assessing all available information and how this would be applied to each patient, balanced by the clinical status and medical co-morbidities of each patient. Targeted therapies can bring new and different sequelae, and oncology teams need to remain fluent in managing the consequences of therapy and primary management. In this book series, we will present how modern care has progressed in multiple disease areas and how modern oncology teams need to adapt in order to manage the cancer patients of today successfully. Surgery, radiation therapy, and medical oncology are practiced today with the support of exceptional modern technology, and in this series, we will review how these improvements are applied to each disease site to maintain excellence in patient care.

# Meet the Series Editor

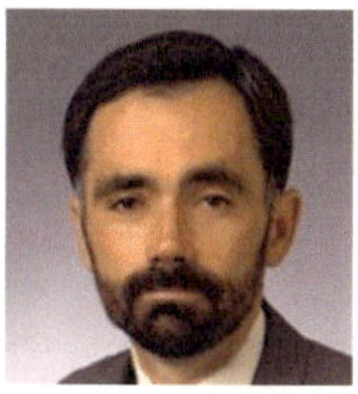

Dr. FitzGerald is the professor and chair of the Department of Radiation Oncology at UMass Chan Medical School in the USA. He serves as one of the principal investigators of the Imaging and Radiation Oncology Core (IROC) service for the National Cancer Institute clinical trials program and is directly involved in the quality assurance of clinical trials in the National Clinical Trials Network (NCTN). Dr. Fitzgerald manages NCTN clinical trials with a real-time pre-therapy review of imaging and radiation therapy treatment objects to ensure the care plan complies with study objectives and the patient stage has been assigned to the correct study. His basic science interest is in hematopoietic stem cell biology and cellular adhesion molecules as they pertain to therapeutic resistance and mitigation of injury from therapy.

# Meet the Volume Editors

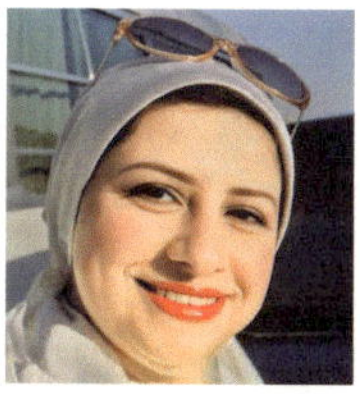

Dr. Marwa Zakaria is a distinguished Professor of Pediatrics, Pediatric Hematology and Oncology at Zagazig University, Egypt. An internationally recognized physician-scientist, she has advanced training from institutions including the European Hematology Association, the Royal Free London NHS Trust, and Boston University. A recipient of the SIOP Award (2018), she is an active member of global societies like SIOP and EHA. Dr. Zakaria has authored over 60 international publications, serves as an Academic Editor, and contributes to national clinical guidelines. She is a sought-after speaker and sub-investigator in international clinical trials, dedicated to advancing care for children with blood disorders and cancer.

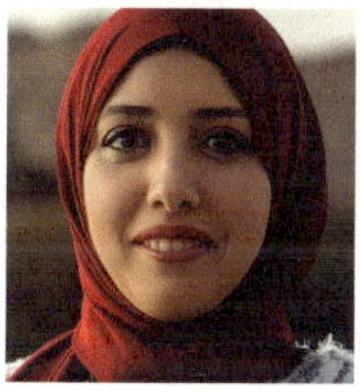

Dr. Samar Elbahy is an Associate Professor of Paediatrics and Paediatric Haematology at Benha University and a Consultant at Benha Children's Hospital in Egypt. A paediatric hematology specialist with 15 years' experience, she holds an MD and completed prestigious international clinical fellowships in paediatric hematology and bone marrow transplantation at Royal Manchester Children's Hospital and Addenbrooke's Hospital, UK, supported by a Newton-Musharafa scholarship. Her research was recognized with the Best Young Abstract Award at EBMT 2019. Dr. Elbahy is an active researcher, guest speaker, and member of clinical committees, and has contributed to numerous publications in paediatric haematology and oncology.

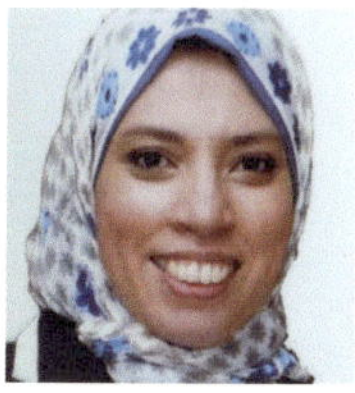

Dr. Al Zahraa Allam is an Associate Professor of Internal Medicine and Hematology at Tanta University, Egypt, with over two decades of clinical and academic experience. An MD and Master's degree holder in Hematology, she currently serves as an adult hematology consultant. Dr. Allam is an active member of several international societies, including the European Hematology Association (EHA) and the European Society for Paediatric Haematology and Oncology (ESPHO). She contributes to her field through extensive research, with over 30 international publications and 15 conference abstracts, and is a frequent guest speaker at national and international hematology forums. Her clinical leadership extends to membership on the Haematology committee at Tanta Insurance Clinic.

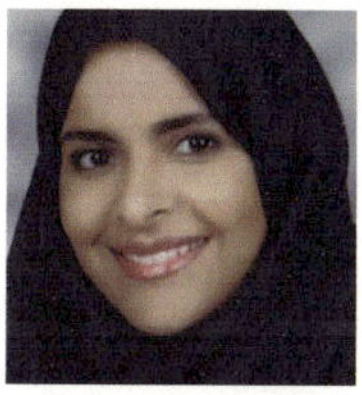

Dr. Hanan Yousif Al-Abboh is a consultant of the Pediatric Hematology Unit at Mubarak Al-Kabeer Hospital in Kuwait. A graduate of Kuwait University's Faculty of Medicine, she completed her pediatric residency and Kuwait Board certification at Mubarak Hospital. She specialized in pediatric hematology under the mentorship of Professor Adekale Kunle, managing a broad spectrum of disorders, including sickle cell disease, thalassemia, hemophilia, and bone marrow failure syndromes. Her advanced training includes an attachment at Cincinnati Children's Hospital in the USA. Actively involved in clinical research, Dr. Al-Abboh is a co-author of several published papers and contributes to postgraduate medical education as a clinical tour instructor for the Kuwait Institution of Medical Specialties.

# Contents

# Preface

The landscape of leukaemia research and clinical practice is transforming more profoundly and rapidly than at any point in its history. What was once a uniformly dire diagnosis has fragmented into a spectrum of distinct diseases, each with its own molecular signature, prognostic profile, and, increasingly, its own tailored therapeutic pathway. This era of unprecedented discovery, fueled by leaps in genomics, immunology, and biotechnology, has fundamentally altered our approach to these complex haematological malignancies. It is within this context of dynamic change that *Leukaemia - Recent Advances in Diagnosis and Therapeutic Modalities* is presented.

This volume was conceived with a clear purpose: to synthesize the cascade of groundbreaking developments from the laboratory bench to the patient's bedside into a coherent, authoritative, and practical resource. We move beyond the foundations to focus squarely on the innovations reshaping the field. From the refined application of next-generation sequencing and minimal residual disease monitoring that guide precision diagnostics, to the revolutionary advent of immunotherapy, CAR T-cell therapy, and novel targeted agents that have redefined treatment paradigms, this book aims to capture the current state of the art.

Our contributing authors, leading clinicians and scientists in their respective domains, have distilled complex data into accessible chapters. They explore not only the remarkable successes but also the ongoing challenges, managing resistance, mitigating novel toxicities, and ensuring equitable access to these advanced modalities. This book is intended for haematologists, oncologists, translational researchers, and senior students who seek a focused update on the forces driving modern leukaemia care.

Ultimately, this compilation is a testament to the collaborative spirit of science and medicine. It reflects a shared commitment to converting scientific insight into tangible hope. As we stand at this pivotal juncture, this book serves as both a snapshot of remarkable progress and a guidepost for the future, dedicated to the patients whose resilience inspires the pursuit of every advance chronicled within these pages.

**Marwa Zakaria**
Professor of Pediatrics,
Faculty of Medicine,
Zagazig University,
Zagazig, Egypt.

**Samar Elbahy**
Associate Professor of Pediatrics,
Faculty of Medicine,
Benha University,
Banha, Egypt

**Al Zahraa Allam**
Associate Professor of Internal Medicine and Hematology,
Tanta University,
Tanta, Egypt

**Hanan Yousif Al-Abboh**
Consultant,
Pediatric Hematology Mubarak Al-Kabeer Hospital,
Jabriya, Kuwait

Chapter 1

# Perspective Chapter: Cutting-Edge Genomic Technologies in the Field of Cancer Cytogenetics

*Shivani Golem*


## Abstract

Optical genome mapping (OGM), with its high resolution and comprehensive analysis of structural and copy number abnormalities, is revolutionizing the field of cancer cytogenomics. Traditional conventional cytogenetics or karyotyping and fluorescent in situ hybridization are the standard-of-care (SOC) assays in cytogenetic laboratory testing for patient care. Chromosomal microarray analysis (CMA), which offers higher resolution than SOC methods, has been widely adopted in many clinical genetics laboratories. It has the caveat of being unable to detect balanced structural rearrangements, and OGM is still developing for detecting copy-neutral loss-of-heterozygosity, which is part of the recurrent genetic abnormalities in many cancer types, including both hematologic malignancies and solid tumor cancer types. The World Health Organization (WHO), National Comprehensive Cancer Network (NCCN), International Consensus Classification (ICC), and many other international organizations have revised, year after year, the guidelines for detecting genomic alterations in several cancers, which help in diagnosis, risk stratification, and treatment management for patients. The number of such genetic abnormalities continues to grow. Therefore, it is imperative to identify such clinically relevant genomic alterations at the gene level, which is possible with CMA and OGM technologies. This chapter will provide a general overview of how cutting-edge technologies complement traditional cytogenetic methods, along with a few case examples to show the need for incorporating high-resolution whole-genome cytogenomic testing in day-to-day clinical cancer testing.


**Keywords:** optical genome mapping, karyotyping, FISH, structural variants, copy number variants, chromosomal microarray, copy-neutral loss-of-heterozygosity (CN-LOH)

## 1. Introduction

In 1956, Tjio and Levan first accurately counted the number of chromosomes [1]. In 1960, the first cancer-causing Philadelphia chromosome abnormality in chronic myeloid leukemia was identified. In 1985, the genes present at the chromosome breakpoints on the 9q and 22q chromosome arms, *ABL1* and *BCR*, were confirmed, respectively, resulting in an oncogenic *BCR::ABL1* gene fusion [1, 2]. Several cancer-related genetic and genomic abnormalities are being discovered every year. The list of these abnormalities, associated with the diagnosis, prognosis, and therapy of patients, is evaluated regularly by national and international workgroups from the World Health Organization (WHO), the National Comprehensive Cancer Network (NCCN), the European Leukemia Network (ELN), the International Consensus Classification (ICC), and other cancer-specific workgroups. Extensive genomic testing is underway in this field, contributing to the discovery of new clinically relevant genetic and genomic abnormalities, as evidenced by the growing number of peer-reviewed publications.

The standard of care (SOC) cytogenetic testing includes chromosome banding analysis (CBA) and fluorescent in situ hybridization (FISH). The next-generation cytogenomic testing includes neoplastic chromosomal microarray (CMA) and optical genome mapping (OGM). Laboratory geneticists specialized in cytogenetics use these tools to identify recurrent and novel genetic and genomic chromosome abnormalities in various hematologic and solid tumor cancers. **Figure 1** illustrates the general steps involved in each technique, from sample collection to data analysis. **Table 1** provides additional preanalytical and analytical parameters, their limitations, and advantages in detecting various genetic and genomic abnormalities, which are biomarkers of the cancer genome.

Conventional cytogenetics, karyotyping, or chromosome band analysis (CBA) is one of the traditional cytogenetic techniques that has been well-established in many laboratories for over five decades. The first cancer cytogenetic abnormality was detected in 1916. This included a 9;22 translocation involving the breakpoint cluster (*BCR*) region and ABL kinase (*ABL1*) gene in a chronic myeloid leukemia patient. Numerous recurrent genetic abnormalities were detected in subsequent years, which played a transformative role in how hematological neoplasms were subtyped, risk-stratified, and treated. This technique has low resolution (~5 Mb) and is labor-intensive, with a high turnaround time (TAT) of 7 to 21 days. For decades, the analysis part of the karyotyping workflow remained unchanged. A very recent advancement was noted with artificial intelligence (AI)-associated karyotyping. This analytical improvement has been shown to reduce analysis time by approximately 50% and improve the detection of abnormal chromosomes [3]. Chromosome band analysis has the advantage of providing a whole-genome genetic profile and can detect a variety of recurrent genetic structural chromosome abnormalities present in cancer genomes, such as balanced/unbalanced translocations, inversions, insertions, mosaicism, and ploidy changes; however, it operates at a low resolution of ~ 5 Mb. **Figure 2a** shows the normal male karyotype, and **Figure 2b** shows the *KMT2A* (11q23) and *MLLT3* (9p21) translocation in an acute myeloid leukemia patient. CBA cannot provide gene-level resolution and may overlook cryptic structural chromosome abnormalities, which include focal gene deletions, duplications, and gene rearrangements that could involve cancer genes.

Fluorescent in situ hybridization, a second common technique extensively used in cytogenetics laboratories, is based on detecting targeted genetic abnormalities using different FISH probe designs. The most common FISH probe types used in hematological and solid tumor malignancies include dual-color dual-fusion, break-apart, and enumeration probes. **Figure 1** shows the typical steps involved in FISH processing and analysis. Given its significantly reduced TAT of approximately 6 ~ 24 hours, this test is preferred for identifying chromosome abnormalities for immediate

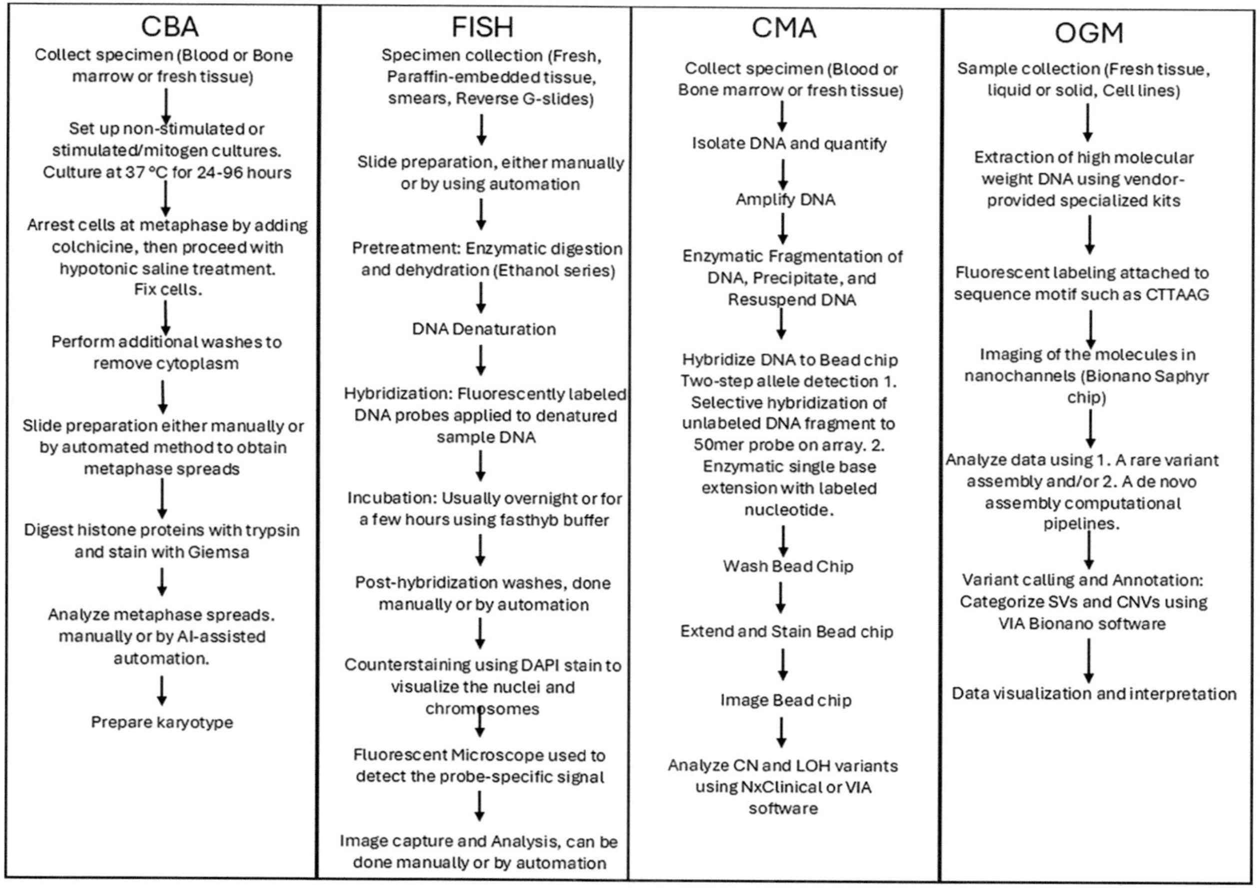


**Figure 1.**
*General overview of the steps involved in the processing of cancer samples for chromosome banding analysis (CBA), FISH, chromosomal microarray analysis (CMA) using the infinium global diversity array (Illumina), and optical genome mapping (OGM) using the Saphyr bionano system. These are not a comprehensive list of steps.*

| Parameters | CBA | FISH | CMA | OGM | Comments |
|---|---|---|---|---|---|
| **Acceptable cancer specimen types** | | | | | |
| >Fresh tissue | TRUE | TRUE | TRUE | TRUE | |
| >Fixed tissue | X | TRUE | TRUE | X | |
| Required DNA concentration | X | X | 150 ng non-FFPE; 400 ng FFPE | 15 μg* | *15 micrograms of ultra-high molecular weight DNA [47]. |
| Processing time | 24-96 hours | 4 hours-1 day | 3 days | 3 days | |
| Analysis time* | 3-7.5 hours | <60 minutes | <60 minutes | 30-120 minutes | Analysis time may vary if the sample has complex genomic abnormalities [24]. |
| Turnaround time | 5-14 days | 6 hours-1 day | 5-10 days | 5-10 days | [24]. |
| **Detection** | | | | | |
| Resolution | 5-10 Mb | 100 kb | 15-200 kb | 500 bp to 1 Mbp* | *[24]. |
| Gene level resolution | X | TRUE | TRUE | TRUE | FISH is limited by probe coverage and requires prior knowledge of the gene(s). |
| **Balanced rearrangements** | | | | | |
| > Translocations | TRUE | TRUE | X | TRUE | |
| >>Balanced whole-arm translocations | TRUE | X | X | X | *[24]. |
| >>End-to-end telomere fusions | TRUE | X | X | X | *[24]. |
| >>Novel balanced translocations | TRUE | X | X | TRUE | |
| >>Cryptic balanced translocations | X | TRUE | X | TRUE | #FISH is limited by probe coverage and requires prior knowledge of the SV and genes. |
| >>Novel intrachromosal deletion translocations | X | X | TRUE | TRUE | |

| Parameters | CBA | FISH | CMA | OGM | Comments |
|---|---|---|---|---|---|
| ≫Cryptic intrachromosal deletion translocations | X | TRUE | TRUE | TRUE | # |
| > Insertion | TRUE | X | X | TRUE | |
| >Inversion | TRUE | TRUE | X | TRUE | # |
| **Unbalanced structural changes** | | | | | |
| >Deletions/ duplications | TRUE | TRUE | TRUE | TRUE | |
| >Partial tandem duplications (PTDs) | X | X | TRUE | TRUE | PTD detected by CMA cannot determine its tandem orientation, for KMT2A PTD. |
| >Gene amplifications | X | TRUE | TRUE | TRUE | |
| Novel unbalanced SVs | TRUE | X | TRUE | TRUE | CMA cannot determine the novel structural chromosomal architecture. |
| Cryptic unbalanced SVs | X | TRUE | TRUE | TRUE | FISH detection is limited by the targeted probe coverage; CMA cannot determine the novel structural chromosome architecture. |
| Map gained genetic material (including marker chromosomes). | X | X | X | TRUE | [21]. |
| > **Complex** | TRUE | X | TRUE | TRUE | CBA – Three or more chromosome abnormalities; Gene level resolution not possible. CMA – SV characterization not possible. |
| Chromoanagenesis | | | | | |
| ≫Chromothripsis | X | X | TRUE | TRUE | |
| ≫Chromoplexy | X | X | X | TRUE | |
| ≫Chromoanasynthesis | X | X | X | TRUE | |
| **LOH** | | | | | |
| ≫Copy Loss – Loss-of-Heterozygosity (CL-LOH) | TRUE | TRUE | TRUE | TRUE | |

| Parameters | CBA | FISH | CMA | OGM | Comments |
|---|---|---|---|---|---|
| ≫Copy Neutral – Loss-of-Heterozygosity (CN-LOH) | X | X | TRUE | * | *LOH detection by OGM is limited to whole-arm or whole-chromosome regions. |
| **Mosaicism and Ploidy** | | | | | |
| ≫Mosaicism detection % | ~14% | 5% | 10-20% | 20%** | OGM – 5% (Rare variant assembly); 15%–25% De novo assembly [24], ** [47]. |
| ≫Ploidy (entire chromosome set) | TRUE | X | * | ** | *3 n; **OGM has to rely on CBA or CMA data to make ploidy calls. CBA might be indicated for those OGM cases with unusual aneuploidy and high variant allele fractions for SVs [24]. |
| ≫Ploidy (single chromosome) | TRUE | TRUE | TRUE | TRUE | |
| **Others** | | | | | |
| ≫Resolve clonal evolution/structure | TRUE | TRUE | X | X | #CMA and OGM have limitations due to bulk DNA genomic analysis. |
| ≫Methylation Profiling | X | X | X | X | |
| ≫Single nucleotide variant detection | X | X | X | X | |
| ≫Minimal residual disease (MRD) detection | TRUE | TRUE | X | X | CMA and OGM testing are recommended at diagnosis and relapse. |
| ≫Cost | $50 | $50-150 | $250-550 | $450-550 | [24]. |
| ≫Bioinformatics | X | X | X | X | |

**Table 1.**
*CBA, FISH, CMA, and OGM testing parameters, genetic abnormality detection characteristics, and limitations.*

treatment decisions, as warranted for specific cancer types. An example is the detection of the *PML::RARA* gene rearrangement in the diagnosis and treatment of acute promyelocytic leukemia. **Figure 2c–e** shows the common FISH probe types used in cancer cytogenetic laboratories and their typical abnormal signal patterns. Comprehensive genomic analysis of the cancer genome is not possible using FISH technology, and the FISH probe coverage for specific target regions limits its detection of genetic abnormalities.

Chromosomal microarray analysis is a long-standing technology that has been used clinically since the mid-2000s for its ability to provide comprehensive genome-wide genetic analysis of both hematologic malignancies and solid tumors [4–9].

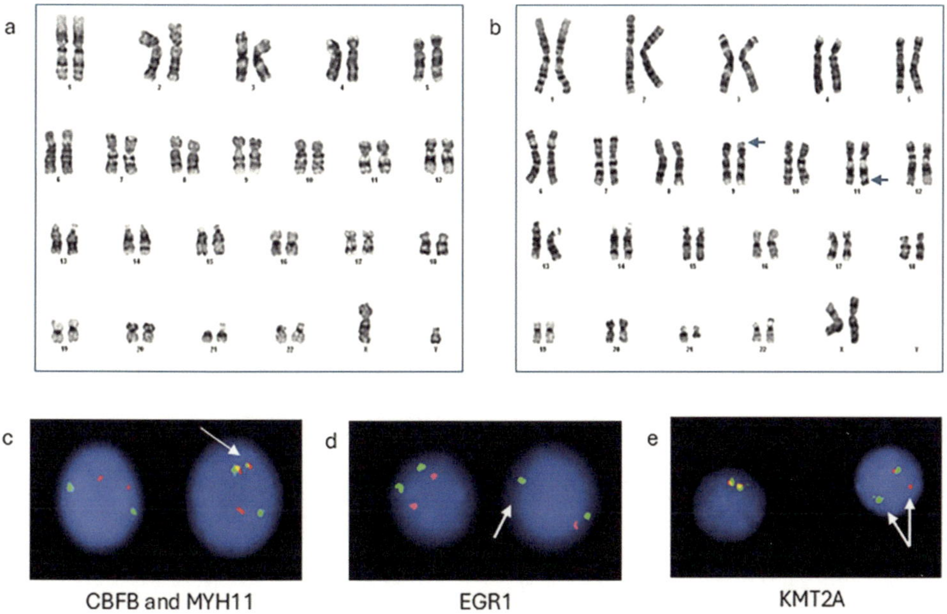


**Figure 2.**
*(a) Karyotype of a normal male chromosome complement; (b) t(9;11)(p21;q23) as indicated by arrows in a female patient with acute myeloid leukemia; (c-e) FISH signal patterns in interphase cells for the most commonly used FISH probes in hematologic cancer, the normal (left) and abnormal (right) cells; (c) the dual-color dual-fusion FISH probe covering the* CBFB *(red) and* MYH11 *(green) gene targets; (d) the deletion FISH probe covering the* EGR1 *(red) and control (green) probes on chromosome 5; (e) the dual-color breakapart FISH probe covering the* KMT2A *gene target. Arrows indicate abnormal FISH signal patterns associated with each of the probe types.*

Chromosomal microarray analysis detects copy number variants (CNVs) (deletions and duplications) and copy-neutral loss-of-heterozygosity (CN-LOH) changes in cancer specimens, along with cryptic deletions and duplications, which the CBA misses. Chromosomal microarray analysis, compared to SOC techniques, detects genetic changes at the gene level more effectively and efficiently, providing a more precise definition of the cancer genome, which is well supported by published literature, including national and international guidelines [10–12]. However, CMA cannot detect balanced structural chromosome abnormalities, such as balanced translocations, insertions, and inversions, which are recurrent genetic abnormalities found in a variety of cancers. Additionally, CMA cannot determine the clonal architecture of the genome.

OGM is revolutionizing the cytogenomics community with its ability to detect comprehensive genome-wide structural variants (SV) and CNVs at high resolution in both constitutional and cancer patient populations [13–24]. OGM can better characterize and refine the complex cancer genome architecture with unbalanced, balanced, and unknown genomic material (marker) chromosome abnormalities [21, 25]. The unique OGM technique allows for this functionality, which could be challenging to detect by CBA due to low resolution, not possible by CMA to refine structural chromosome changes and detect balanced genomic alterations, and by FISH due to the limitation of the need for prior knowledge of the gene targets and the lack of comprehensive whole genome assessment.

## 2. Structural and copy number variants

Multiple studies have shown high concordance between CMA and OGM in detecting copy number variants in both hematologic and solid tumor malignancies compared to SOC methods. **Figure 3** illustrates some case examples where OGM detected cryptic deletions that CBA missed. An apparently balanced translocation of 2;4 by karyotype (**Figure 3a, b**) revealed a cryptic *DNMT3A* gene deletion at the 2p23 translocation breakpoint, which was detected by OGM (**Figure 3c**). A similar case example of an apparent 1;7 translocation showed a cryptic *IKZF1* gene deletion at the 7p translocation breakpoint, identified by CMA (**Figure 4a–c**). Both examples highlight the limitations of CBA in detecting these clinically relevant gene deletions, which are of prognostic significance [26]. In another case, the *TET2* gene was disrupted due to an intragenic cryptic inversion of 4q24q24, detected by OGM (**Figure 3d**). Chromosomal Microarray Analysis would miss this balanced intragenic inversion event. This case example underscores the limitations of CMA in detecting balanced structural abnormalities of the genome. A 20q11.21q11.22 deletion, 2 Mb in size and involving the clinically relevant gene *ASXL1* (**Figure 3e**), as well as a 1 Mb Xp11.4 deletion involving the *BCOR* cancer-relevant gene (**Figure 3f**) were detected by OGM and can also be detected by CMA (not shown in the image) [26]. Both CMA and OGM are capable of detecting similar unbalanced deletions and duplications, subject to their size detection limitations/resolution (**Table 1**).

The t(6;9)(p22;q34) *DEK::NUP214* gene rearrangement is a chromosomal abnormality that has been identified in approximately 1% of myelodysplastic neoplasms and acute myeloid leukemias. The t(6;9) is also frequently associated with basophilia and is generally considered a poor-risk acute myeloid leukemia (AML) subgroup [27, 28]. Although t(6;9) is visible by CBA, there are reported cases, such as an AML case with a t(9;12)(q34;q15) karyotype and normal morphology for the 6p region. RNA-sequencing confirmed a cryptic *DEK::NUP214* fusion [29]. Another case of AML with an original karyotype of add(6)(p21), add(9)(q34), add(14)(q22) was suspicious of a 6;9 translocation with 6p21 and 9q34 breakpoints and a *DEK::NUP214* fusion; FISH on an abnormal metaphase was performed. FISH confirmed *DEK* and *NUP214* signals on the abnormal chromosome 6, which confirmed the *DEK::NUP214* fusion. Based on the FISH results, the karyotype was updated to t(6;14;9)(p22;q22; q34). The OGM performed on this sample confirmed the FISH result with a three-way translocation and confirmed in-frame *DEK* gene alignment with the *NUP214* gene on the abnormal chromosome 6 [30]. In another myeloid neoplasm case, CBA detected a 48,XY, +8, +9, t(9;9)(p21;q12) karyotype (**Figure 5a**), 5'*PDGFRβ* deletion by interphase FISH (**Figure 5b**), and a cryptic deletion of 5q32q32.1 of < 1 Mb in size by CMA (**Figure 5c**). A zoomed-in **Figure 5c** image shows that the deletion encompasses the 5' region of the *PDGFRβ* gene as well as 19 other RefSeq genes, including the 3'*TNIP1* gene deletion, and this intrachromosomal deletion is expected to result in *TNIP1::PDGFRβ* gene fusion. The *PDGFRβ* gene retains the catalytic domain (exons 13–21) of the *PDGFRβ* protein [31]. This result is consistent with the diagnosis of myeloid neoplasms associated with *PDGFRβ* rearrangement per the WHO classification of cancer subtypes. A tyrosine kinase inhibitor can target *PDGFRβ* rearrangement. These case examples demonstrate how CMA and OGM can identify clinically significant cryptic fusions, thereby changing patient therapy management based on the findings. These cases also highlight limitations and the necessity for additional tests, such as FISH, to validate karyotype findings. Given that CMA can

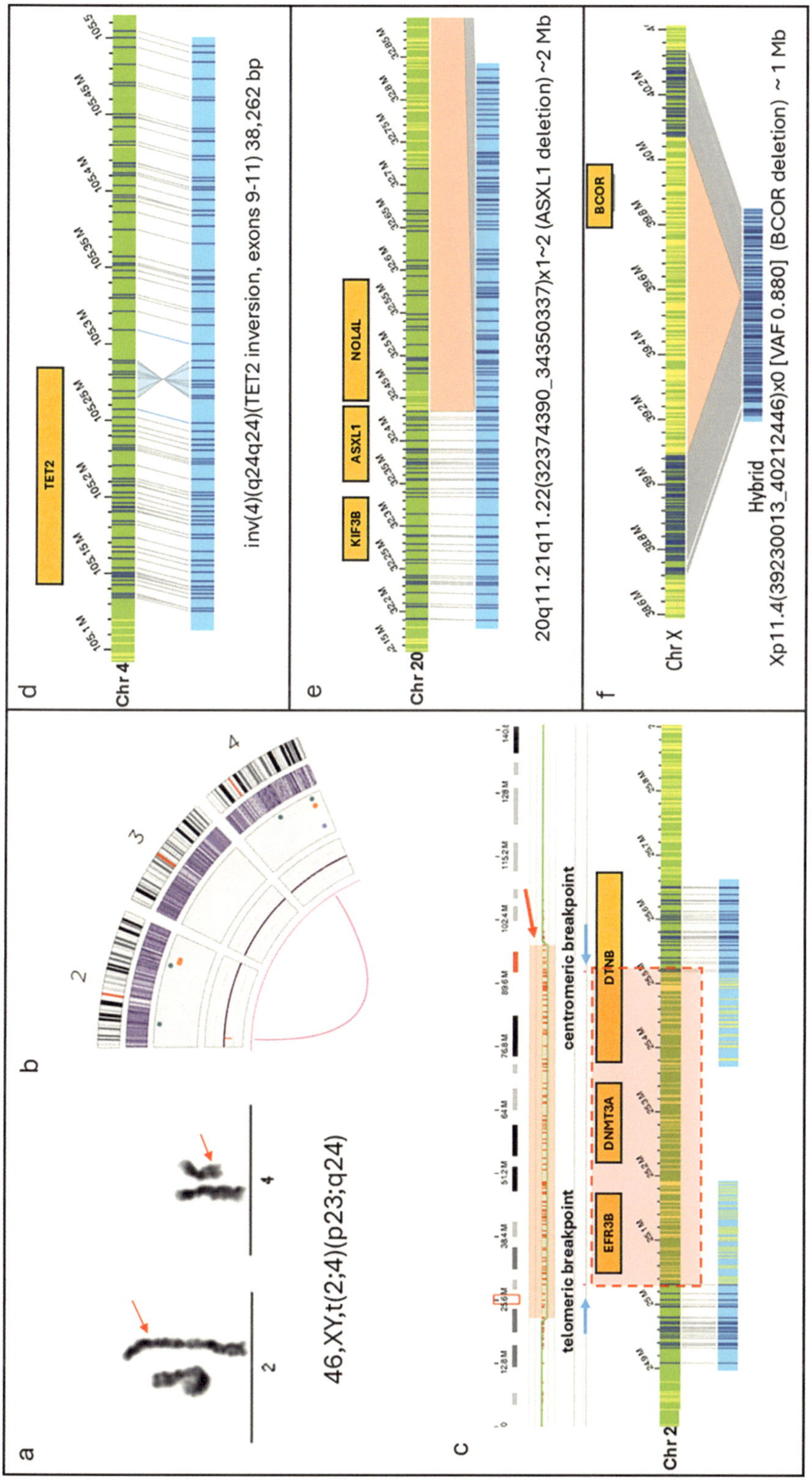


**Figure 3.**
*Images show the SVS detected by OGM that are missed by karyotyping, which are of diagnostic and therapeutic significance for patients. (a) Partial karyotype with apparent balanced t(2;4)(p23;q24). (b) OGM circus plot showing similar t(2;4) indicated by the magenta line connecting chromosomes 2 and 4. (c) High-resolution view of the chromosome 2 breakpoint shows an interstitial deletion involving* EFR3B, DNMT3A, *and* DTNB *genes. See additional description in the original open-access article [26]. (d) Intragenic inversion involving the* TET2 *gene's exons 9–11 of 38 kb in size is shown. (e) A 2 Mb deletion on chromosome 20q is shown, which includes the* ASXL1 *gene. (f) A 1 Mb deletion on Xp involving the* BCOR *gene is shown. The figure is reproduced with permission from Dr. Adam C. Smith, University of Toronto, Toronto, Canada, and Dr. Gordana Raca, Children's Hospital Los Angeles, Los Angeles, USA, from their open-access published article [26].*

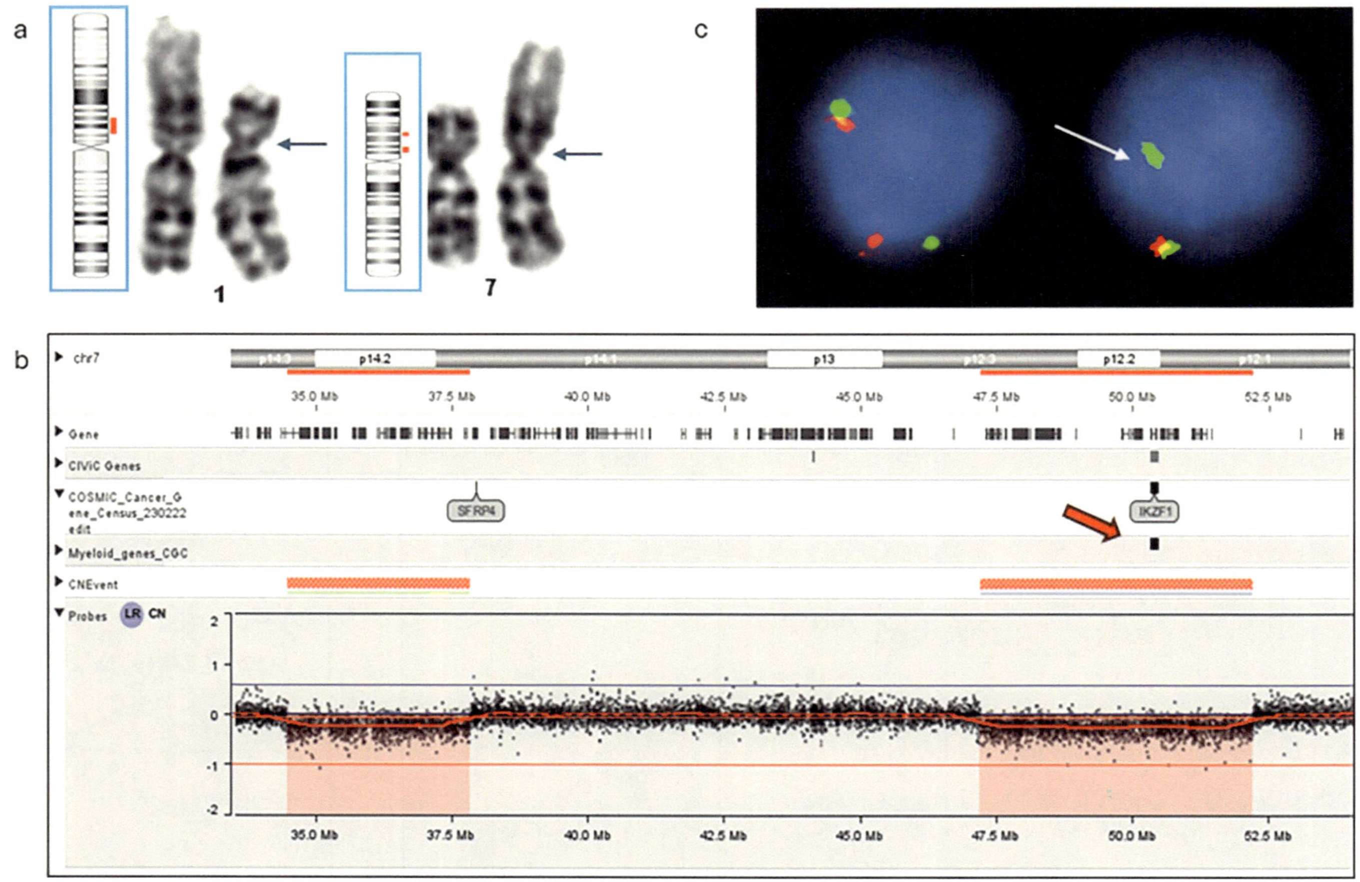


**Figure 4.**
*A case of AML evolved from a CML with a karyotype of 46,XX,t(9;22)(q34;q11.2)[4]/46,sl,t(1;7)(p11;p11.2)[16]. (a) Partial karyotype of the subclone showing an apparent balanced translocation of 1;7, indicated by arrows. The blue box displays the CMA partial virtual karyotype with losses (red bars) on the 1p and 7p translocation chromosome arms. (b) CMA data shows a telomeric 3.4 Mb deletion of 7124.3P14.1, and a centromeric 5 Mb deletion of 7p12.3p12.1, which includes the* IKZF1 *clinically relevant gene deletion (red arrow), which was missed by karyotype. (c) Interphase FISH shows the* IKZF1 *(red) deletion, shown by the white arrow.*

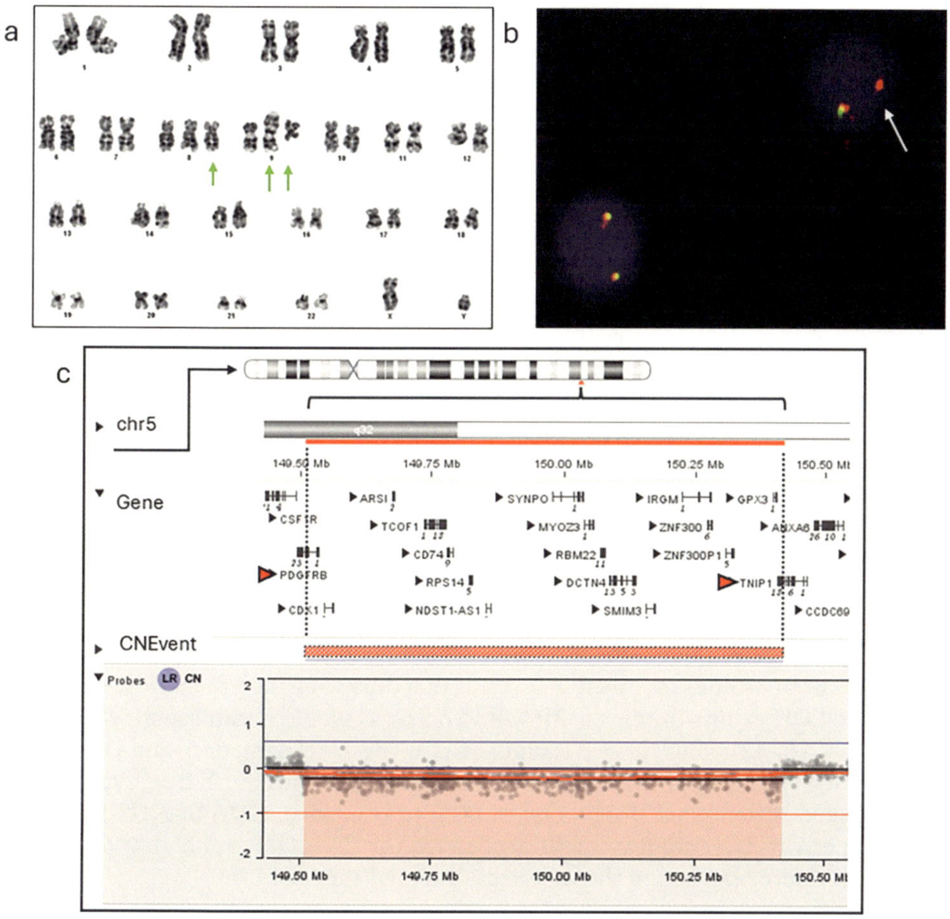


**Figure 5.**
*(a) Chromosome G-band image showing a 48,XY,+8,+9,t(9;9)(p21;q12) karyotype. The arrow indicates an abnormal chromosome. (b)* PDGFRB *breakapart FISH shows intact gene signals with 3' (red) and 5' (green) fused signals in the normal nuclei (left) and deletion of the green 5'* PDGFRB *signal in an abnormal nucleus (right, white arrow). (c) CMA result showing chromosome 5 with a < 1 Mb (911 kb) deletion of 5q32.1. The proximal and distal breakpoints of the deletion include* PDGFRB *and* TNIP1 *genes, shown as dashed lines and boxes, respectively. This intrachromosomal deletion results in a* TNIP1::PDGFRB *fusion.*

detect intrachromosomal deletions and their associated gene fusions but will miss balanced gene fusions, OGM in such scenarios would be a better option to characterize these cryptic and complex balanced and unbalanced fusions at the gene-level resolution without any additional ancillary testing needs.

## 3. Copy-neutral loss-of-heterozygosity

Copy-neutral loss-of-heterozygosity is defined as the loss of a copy of an allele and the duplication of the remaining allele, which results in two copies of the same allele, known as uniparental disomy. This is an essential and common cancer biomarker that could unmask recessive mutations or enhance oncogene expression. CMA has proven to be a reliable test in detecting prognostically important CN-LOH events, including the 13q chromosome region encompassing the *FLT3* gene and the

17p region encompassing the *TP53* gene in AML [32]. According to recent updates of the WHO classification of myeloid neoplasms, CN-LOH involving the *TP53* gene, along with a *TP53* variant, would identify MDS diagnostic criteria as "MDS with biallelic *TP53* inactivation" or "MDS with mutated *TP53*" [33, 34]. OGM does not employ single-nucleotide polymorphism (SNP) analysis, a crucial tool for detecting CN-LOH. Consequently, current LOH detection is restricted to either the entire chromosome or a specific chromosome arm. This limitation could significantly affect the detection of clinically relevant and prognostically important focal CN-LOH biomarkers that cover cancer genes, such as *TP53, FLT3, RB1, JAK2, WT1, CEBPA, RUNX1,* and *TET2* [35–37], which provide a growth advantage to cancer cells. Detection of these CN-LOH events in these clinically relevant cancer genes could change the prognostic risk group and patient management. The diagnostic challenge of differentiating bone marrow features of acquired aplastic anemia, hypocellular MDS, and inherited bone marrow failure is critical in selecting appropriate therapy. The presence of CN-LOH on the 6p chromosome, which can occur in focal LOH events, has been shown to favor a diagnosis of aplastic anemia. Copy-neutral loss-of-heterozygosity detection testing is indicated in such scenarios [38–40]. OGM is still developing techniques to identify CN-LOH, making it unavailable for detecting these important cancer biomarkers, which CMA can detect [20].

In B-cell acute lymphoblastic leukemia (ALL), proper characterization of a seemingly hyperdiploid clone as doubled-hypodiploid by detecting the CN-LOH for those chromosomes involved will result in a drastic change in clinical outcomes. These CN-LOH events in this entity would occur as whole chromosome events. A SNP-based CMA, which is well established for CN-LOH detection, and OGM using the De Novo Assembly pipeline for LOH detection, can distinguish true hyperdiploid from masked hypodiploid B-ALL clones [41]. In summary, CMA or NGS-based detection of CN-LOH studies is still needed for the CN-LOH events that occur as focal LOH and/or fall below the detection limits of the OGM.

## 4. Complex chromosome abnormalities and chromoanagenesis

Complex karyotypes are a common finding in cancers and indicate genomic instability. The presence of three or more chromosome abnormalities is traditionally considered complex. CBA has been widely used for identifying complex structural and numerical genomic changes for over five decades. However, due to its low resolution, the detection of complexity and the genes affected in such abnormalities was limited, which was addressed with the implementation of CMA. CMA was able to identify cryptic CNVs, which helped in re-stratifying the prognostic risk for cancer patients. CMA cannot detect balanced structural changes, which are an integral part of cancer-associated genetic changes, and these are missed. The OGM was able to close the gap in this limitation by detecting both the CNVs and SVs associated with the complex cancer genome. The prognostic significance of complex karyotype, defined as the presence of three unrelated clonal changes, is well known for its association with very poor outcomes and even higher relapse rates following transplant [42].

The complexity of the cancer genome was further defined by chromoanagenesis, which encompasses complex genomic alterations. Chromoanagenesis includes chromothripsis, chromoplexy, and chromoanasynthesis genomic alterations. These complex chromosomal rearrangements happen in a single cell cycle and indicate genomic instability. Chromothripsis involves the clustered shattering of the genome, followed by random reassembly. Chromoplexy, on the other hand, involves multiple sequential translocations across multiple chromosomes, all occurring in a single catastrophic event. Additionally, chromoanasynthesis involves DNA replication errors due to replication stress factors, which result in the clustered presence of CN changes (gains and losses) and CN-LOH events [43]. These genetic changes are reported in multiple other cancer types, including multiple myeloma [44], CLL [45], and AML [46]. **Figure 6** shows the complex genomic changes with SVs and CNVs (**Figure 6a, b**) detected by OGM, along with a chromothripsis of chromosome 2 (**Figure 6c**). The OGM helps resolve and better characterize the structural and copy number abnormalities detected by karyotype [23]. Chromoanagenesis has been associated with poor outcomes, with extensive clonal heterogeneity and refractory disease in AML [46]. Similar complex genomes with CNVs and CN-LOH events are also detected by the CMA, including chromothripsis events, as shown in (**Figure 7a–c**). Data analysis by CBA or FISH is labor-intensive without automation or AI assistance technology. The CMA or OGM analysis is not time-consuming when the genomic profile is not complex; however, when complex genomic alterations are present, it can be challenging. The entire data analysis of the CMA and OGM output is highly visual, simplifying interpretations and analysis, and eliminating the need for a complex bioinformatics pipeline resource, which is used for whole exome and genome sequencing [24]. However, there are also challenges in eliminating false calls, such as balanced translocations called by OGM but not verified by CBA or FISH.

## 5. Novel SVs and CNVs tier classification

Guidelines from the American College of Medical Genetics and Genomics (ACMG) provide a four-tier evidence-based categorization system for acquired CNVs and CN-LOH events detected by CMA, based on the level of evidence supported by the CEBM Oxford Centre for Evidence-Based Medicine, COG (Children's Oncology Group), COSMIC (Catalogue of Somatic Mutations in Cancer), IPSS (International Prognostic Scoring System for myelodysplastic syndromes), NCCN, WHO, and peer-reviewed publications [10]. These include Tier 1: Variants with strong clinical significance, Tier 2: Variants with some clinical significance, Tier 3: Clonal variants with no documented neoplastic disorder association, and Tier 4: Benign or likely benign variants [10]. These guidelines apply to OGM's SVs and CNVs tier classification [47]. However, the limited data on novel OGM findings with unknown oncogenic significance will be triaged as Tier 3. All these novel OGM findings require further studies to better characterize their roles in diagnostic, prognostic, and therapeutic contexts in specific cancer types.

## 6. Clonal architecture

Historically, CBA and FISH analysis have been based on the analysis of single-cell genetic abnormalities and are reported as a proportion of affected cells, which differ significantly from cutting-edge cytogenomic technologies, including CMA, OGM, and next-generation sequencing-based analysis. These newer technologies involve multiple-cell pooled or bulk DNA analysis from a case and are reported as variant

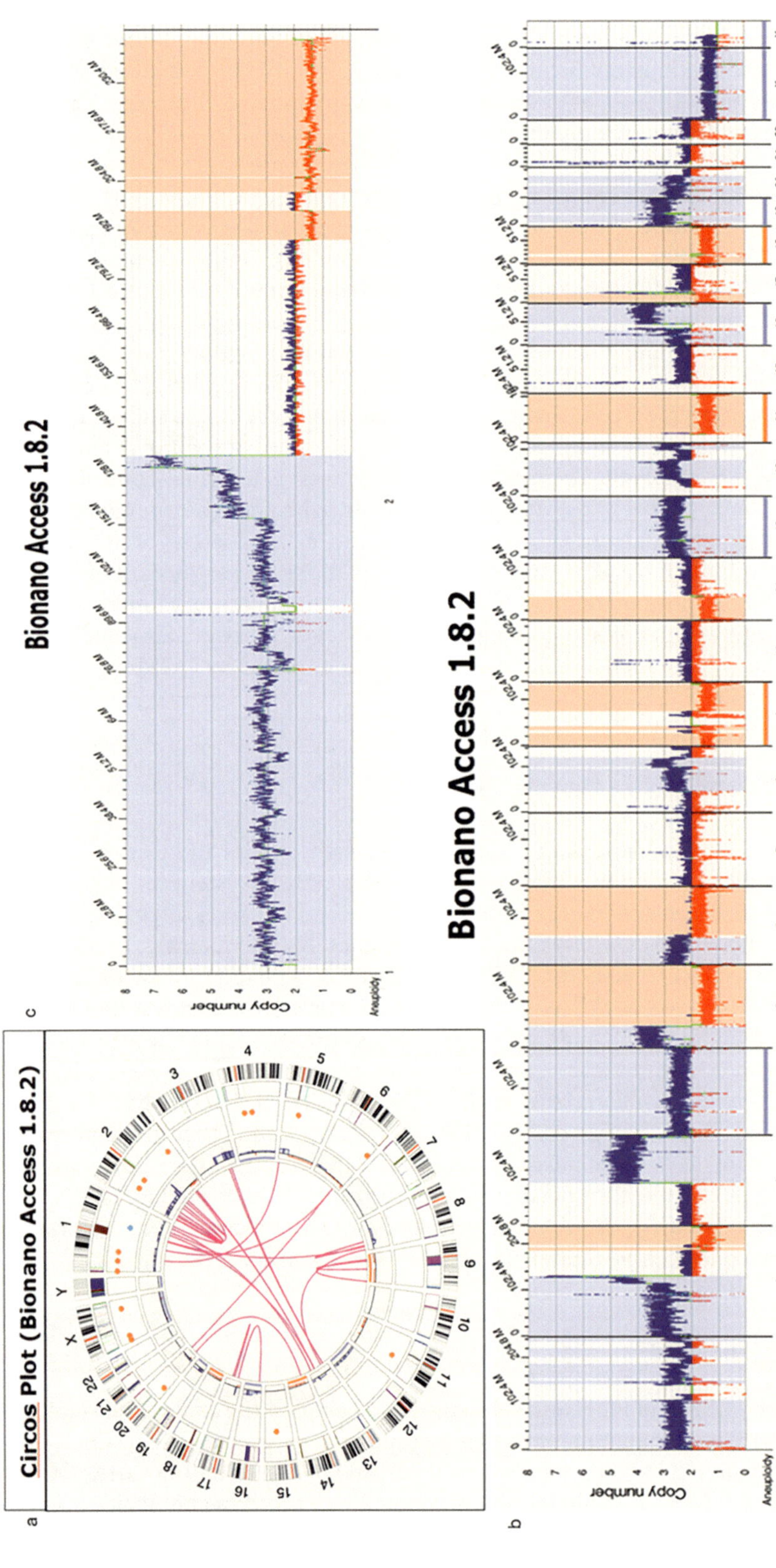


**Figure 6.**
*OGM analysis. The OGM circos plot (a) and whole genome view (b) analysis detected a complex genomic profile with multiple structural changes. (c). OGM technology detected chromothripsis of chromosome 2 with multiple copy number changes with alternating normal CN events. Images are courtesy of Dr. M. Anwar Iqbal, University of Rochester Medical Center, Rochester, NY, USA.*

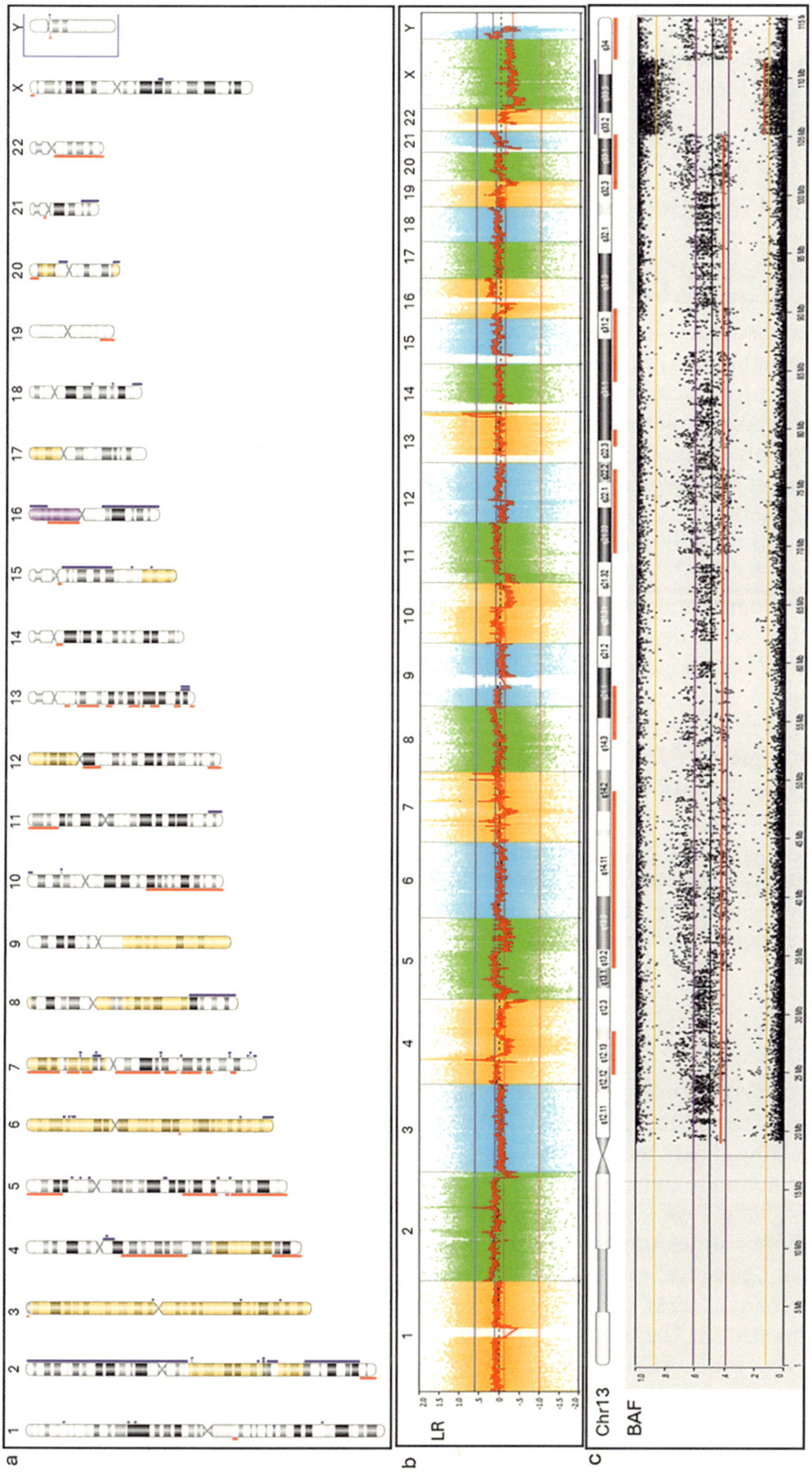


**Figure 7.**
*CMA result showing a complex genomic profile from a male patient with a brain tumor. (a) Virtual karyotype showing blue bars next to chromosomes as gains, red as losses, and yellow as CN-LOH events. (b) Whole genome view based on the log R ratio (LR) view of the same complex genomic profile from a brain tumor case. (c) CMA showing chromothripsis of chromosome 13 from the same case.*

allele fraction (VAF) or copy number alterations, which do not represent cell-level abnormalities but rather are values obtained after data conversion based on the proportion of the sample. This data conversion is further complicated by acquired homozygosity, tumor heterogeneity, and overlapping structural and copy number variants [48].

## 7. Analytical sensitivity and clinical utility

OGM studies are largely focused on hematologic malignancies, including myeloid malignancies, MDS, MPN, MDS/MPN, AML, B-cell ALL, multiple myeloma, and chronic lymphocytic leukemia. This might be due to the need for ultra-high molecular weight DNA, which requires fresh blood and bone marrow samples. OGM cannot be performed on hypocellular samples or fixed cell samples. This greatly limits its universal replacement of CBA, FISH, and CMA tests. Most of the studies published involved comparing OGM to the low-resolution CBA and were mainly limited to myeloid malignancies. Comparison of OGM to all the established cytogenetic methods – CBA, FISH, and CMA – in a large patient population with lymphoma and solid tumor cancer types is limited. There was limited analytical sensitivity and clinical utility of OGM in MPN and MDS/MPN with a normal karyotype in identifying additional abnormalities, except for *KMT2A*-PTD [47]. *KMT2A*-PTD can be detected by currently available CMA (**Figure 8a, b**) [49]; however, the tandem nature of this duplication cannot be determined by CMA.

Although OGM offers whole-genomic SVs and CNVs detection, studies have suggested triaging hematologic malignancies to perform OGM to fully benefit from its use. The clinical utility of OGM differed based on the specific hematologic cancer. Reported clinical utility varies significantly – from 0% to 52% – with the greatest impact observed in B-cell and T-cell malignancies, and more limited utility in myeloid neoplasms, particularly myeloproliferative neoplasms (MPNs) [47]. Larger, well-designed clinical studies are needed to evaluate the clinical utility of OGM across a broad spectrum of myeloid, lymphoid, and solid tumor malignancies, with comprehensive comparisons to CBA, FISH, and CMA methods.

## 8. Conclusion

Comprehensive cancer genome analysis using high-resolution platforms such as chromosomal microarray analysis (CMA) and optical genome mapping (OGM) is rapidly evolving. These technologies complement standard-of-care (SOC) cytogenetic methods and are increasingly being adopted by clinical laboratories. As next-generation cytogenetics tools, CMA and OGM enable detailed assessment of genomic abnormalities across various cancer types, providing insights that are diagnostically, prognostically, and therapeutically significant [4–6, 15–24, 50–55]. Despite their advantages, both advanced and SOC cytogenetic techniques have inherent limitations. Therefore, a strategic and case-specific approach is essential when selecting the most informative assay. This decision should be guided by a thorough evaluation of the cancer type, along with consideration of preanalytical factors, analytical sensitivity, and clinical utility. Such triaging ensures optimal integration of cytogenetic and genomic tools into clinical practice.

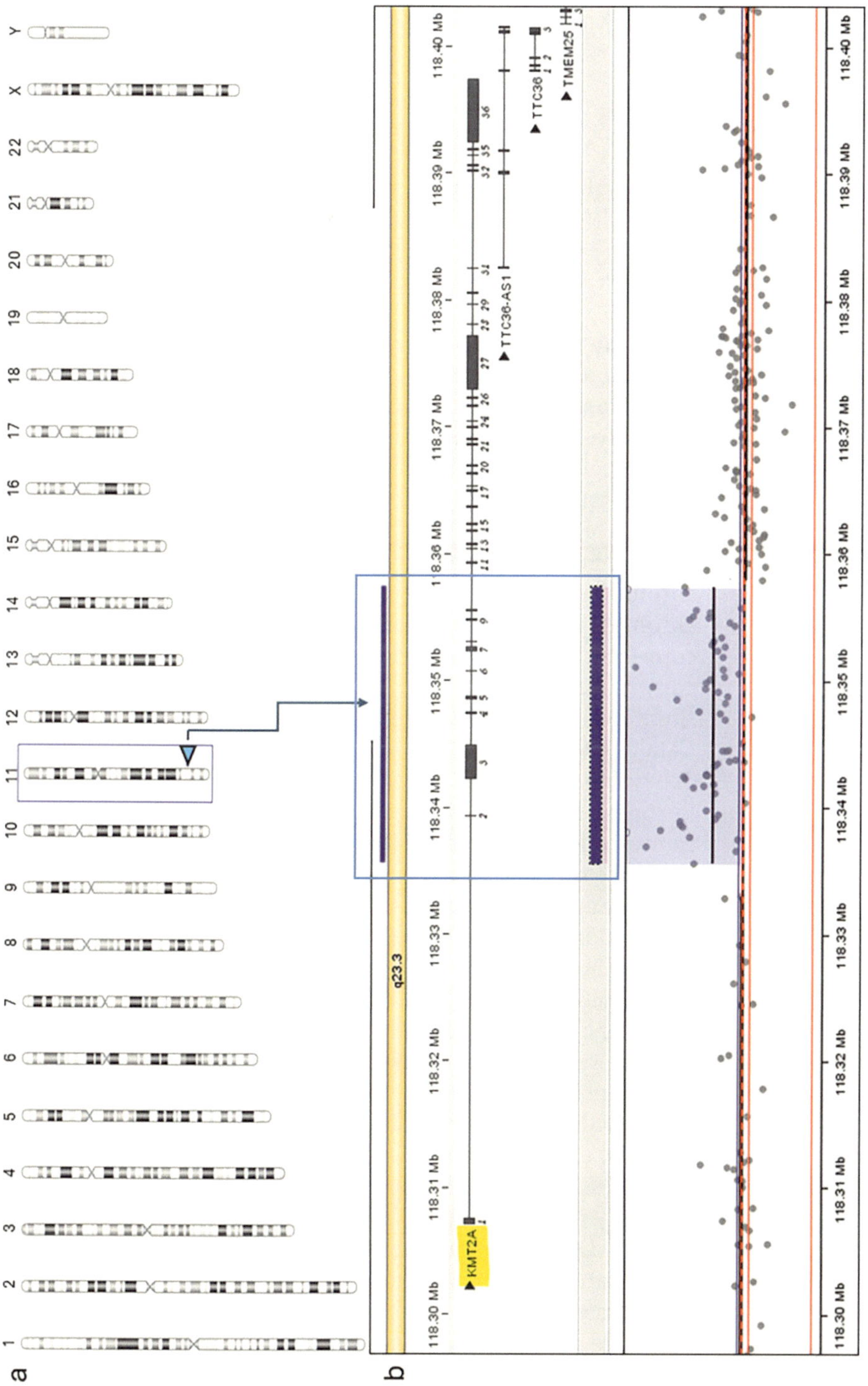


**Figure 8.**
*In an AML patient with a normal karyotype: (a) A virtual karyotype of CMA shows a focal 21 kb region in size on the chromosome 11q arm. (b)* KMT2A *copy gain involving exons 2–10 was detected (blue box).*

## Acknowledgments

The author gratefully acknowledges Drs. Smith, Raca, and Iqbal for generously providing selected images featured in this chapter.

## Conflict of Interest

The author declares no conflict of interest.

## Abbreviations

| | |
|---|---|
| ACMG | American College of Medical Genetics and Genomics |
| AI | artificial intelligence |
| ALL | acute lymphoblastic leukemia |
| AML | acute myeloid leukemia |
| B-ALL | B-cell acute lymphoblastic leukemia |
| CBA | chromosome banding analysis |
| CEBM | Centre for Evidence-Based Medicine (Oxford) |
| CEBPA | CCAAT Enhancer-Binding Protein Alpha |
| CLL | chronic lymphocytic leukemia |
| CMA | chromosomal microarray analysis |
| CN-LOH | copy-neutral loss-of-heterozygosity |
| CNV | copy number variants |
| COG | Children's Oncology Group |
| COSMIC | Catalogue of Somatic Mutations in Cancer |
| DNA | deoxyribonucleic acid |
| ELN | European Leukemia Network |
| FISH | fluorescent in situ hybridization |
| FLT3 | FMS-like tyrosine kinase 3 |
| ICC | International Consensus Classification |
| IPSS | International Prognostic Scoring System |
| JAK2 | Janus Kinase 2 |
| LOH | loss of heterozygosity |
| MDS | myelodysplastic syndrome |
| MDS/MPN | overlap syndrome of myelodysplastic and myeloproliferative neoplasms |
| MPN | myeloproliferative neoplasm |
| NCCN | National Comprehensive Cancer Network |
| NGS | next-generation sequencing |
| OGM | optical genome mapping |
| PDGFRβ | platelet-derived growth factor receptor beta |
| PTD | partial tandem duplication |
| RB1 | retinoblastoma 1 |
| RefSeq | reference sequence database |
| RNA | ribonucleic acid |
| RUNX1 | runt-related transcription factor 1 |
| SNP | single-nucleotide polymorphism |

| | |
|---|---|
| SOC | standard of care |
| SV | structural variants |
| TAT | turnaround time |
| TET2 | TET methylcytosine dioxygenase 2 |
| TNIP1 | TNFAIP1 interacting protein 1 |
| TP53 | tumor protein p53 |
| VAF | variant allele fraction |
| WHO | World Health Organization |
| WT1 | Wilms Tumor 1 |

## Author details

Shivani Golem
University of Kansas Medical Center, Kansas, USA

*Address all correspondence to: sgolem@kumc.edu

## References


[1] Trask BJ. Human cytogenetics: 46 chromosomes, 46 years and counting. Nature Reviews Genetics. 2002;**3** (10):769–778. DOI: 10.1038/nrg905

[2] Heisterkamp N, Stam K, Groffen J, de Klein A, Grosveld G. Structural organization of the BCR gene and its role in the Ph' translocation. Nature. 1985;**315**(6022):758–761. DOI: 10.1038/315758a0

[3] Rosenblum LS, Holmes J, Taghiyev AF. The emergence of artificial intelligence-guided karyotyping: A review and reflection. Genes (Basel). 2025;**16**(6):685. DOI: 10.3390/genes16060685

[4] Chun K, et al. Assessing copy number aberrations and copy-neutral loss-of-heterozygosity across the genome as best practice: An evidence-based review from the cancer genomics consortium (CGC) working group for chronic lymphocytic leukemia. Cancer Genetics. 2018;**228-229**:236–250

[5] Kanagal-Shamanna R, et al. Assessing copy number aberrations and copy neutral loss of heterozygosity across the genome as best practice: An evidence-based review of clinical utility from the cancer genomics consortium (CGC) working group for myelodysplastic syndrome, myelodysplastic/myeloproliferative and myeloproliferative neoplasms. Cancer Genetics. 2018;**228-229**:197–217

[6] Xu X, Bryke C, Sukhanova M, Huxley E, Dash DP, Dixon-Mciver A, Fang M, Griepp PT, Hodge JC, Iqbal A, Jeffries S, Kanagal-Shamanna R, Quintero-Rivera F, Shetty S, Slovak ML, Yenamandra A, Lennon PA, Raca G. Assessing copy number abnormalities and copy-neutral loss-of-heterozygosity across the genome as best practice in diagnostic evaluation of acute myeloid leukemia: An evidence-based review from the cancer genomics consortium (CGC) myeloid neoplasms working group. Cancer Genetics. 2018;**228-229**:218–235. DOI: 10.1016/j.cancergen.2018.07.005

[7] Dougherty MJ, Tooke LS, Sullivan LM, Hakonarson H, Wainwright LM, Biegel JA. Clinical utilization of high-resolution single nucleotide polymorphism based oligonucleotide arrays in diagnostic studies of pediatric patients with solid tumors. Cancer Genetics. 2012;**205** (1-2):42–54. DOI: 10.1016/j.cancergen.2012.01.014

[8] Wang Y, Miller S, Roulston D, Bixby D, Shao L. Genome-wide single-nucleotide polymorphism array analysis improves prognostication of acute lymphoblastic leukemia/lymphoma. Journal of Molecular Diagnostics. 2016;**18**(4):595–603. DOI: 10.1016/j.jmoldx.2016.03.004

[9] Roth JJ, Santi M, Rorke-Adams LB, Harding BN, Busse TM, Tooke LS, Biegel JA. Diagnostic application of high resolution single nucleotide polymorphism array analysis for children with brain tumors. Cancer Genetics. 2014;**207**(4):111–123. DOI: 10.1016/j.cancergen.2014.03.002

[10] Mikhail FM, Biegel JA, Cooley LD, Dubuc AM, Hirsch B, Horner VL, Newman S, Shao L, Wolff DJ, Raca G. Technical laboratory standards for interpretation and reporting of acquired

copy-number abnormalities and copy-neutral loss of heterozygosity in neoplastic disorders: A joint consensus recommendation from the American College of Medical Genetics and Genomics (ACMG) and the Cancer Genomics Consortium (CGC). Genetics in Medicine. 2019;**21**(9):1903–1916. DOI: 10.1038/s41436-019-0545-7

[11] Berry NK, Scott RJ, Rowlings P, Enjeti AK. Clinical use of SNP-microarrays for the detection of genome-wide changes in haematological malignancies. Critical Reviews in Oncology/Hematology. 2019;**142**:58–67. DOI: 10.1016/j.critrevonc.2019.07.016

[12] Shao L, Akkari Y, Cooley LD, Miller DT, Seifert BA, Wolff DJ, Mikhail FM, ACMG Laboratory Quality Assurance Committee. Chromosomal microarray analysis, including constitutional and neoplastic disease applications, 2021 revision: A technical standard of the American College of Medical Genetics and Genomics (ACMG). Genetics in Medicine. 2021;**23** (10):1818–1829. DOI: 10.1038/s41436-021-01214-w

[13] Iqbal MA, Broeckel U, Levy B, Skinner S, Sahajpal NS, Rodriguez V, Stence A, Awayda K, Scharer G, Skinner C, Stevenson R, Bossler A, Nagy PL, Kolhe R. Multisite assessment of optical genome mapping for analysis of structural variants in constitutional postnatal cases. Journal of Molecular Diagnostics. 2023;**25**(3):175–188. DOI: 10.1016/j.jmoldx.2022.12.005

[14] Kanagal-Shamanna R, Puiggros A, Granada I, Raca G, Rack K, Mallo M, Dewaele B, Smith AC, Akkari Y, Levy B, Hasserjian RP, Cisneros A, Salido M, Garcia-Manero G, Yang H, Iqbal MA, Kolhe R, Solé F, Espinet B. Integration of optical genome mapping in the cytogenomic and molecular work-up of hematological malignancies: Expert recommendations from the international consortium for optical genome mapping. American Journal of Hematology. 2025;**100**(6):1029–1048. DOI: 10.1002/ajh.27688

[15] Duncavage EJ, Schroeder MC, O'Laughlin M, Wilson R, MacMillan S, Bohannon A, Kruchowski S, Garza J, Du F, Hughes AEO, Robinson J, Hughes E, Heath SE, Baty JD, Neidich J, Christopher MJ, Jacoby MA, Uy GL, Fulton RS, Miller CA, Payton JE, Link DC, Walter MJ, Westervelt P, DiPersio JF, Ley TJ, Spencer DH. Genome sequencing as an alternative to cytogenetic analysis in myeloid cancers. New England Journal of Medicine. 2021;**384**(10):924–935. DOI: 10.1056/NEJMoa2024534

[16] Yang H, Garcia-Manero G, Sasaki K, Montalban-Bravo G, Tang Z, Wei Y, Kadia T, Chien K, Rush D, Nguyen H, Kalia A, Nimmakayalu M, Bueso-Ramos C, Kantarjian H, Medeiros LJ, Luthra R, Kanagal-Shamanna R. High-resolution structural variant profiling of myelodysplastic syndromes by optical genome mapping uncovers cryptic aberrations of prognostic and therapeutic significance. Leukemia. 2022;**36**(9):2306–2316. DOI: 10.1038/s41375-022-01652-8

[17] Lühmann JL, Stelter M, Wolter M, Kater J, Lentes J, Bergmann AK, Schieck M, Göhring G, Möricke A, Cario G, Žaliová M, Schrappe M, Schlegelberger B, Stanulla M, Steinemann D. The clinical utility of optical genome mapping for the assessment of genomic aberrations in acute lymphoblastic leukemia. Cancers (Basel). 2021;**13**(17):4388. DOI: 10.3390/cancers13174388

[18] Rack K, De Bie J, Ameye G, Gielen O, Demeyer S, Cools J, De Keersmaecker K, Vermeesch JR, Maertens J, Segers H, Michaux L, Dewaele B. Optimizing the diagnostic workflow for acute lymphoblastic leukemia by optical genome mapping. American Journal of Hematology. 2022;**97**(5):548–561. DOI: 10.1002/ajh.26487

[19] Puiggros A, Ramos-Campoy S, Kamaso J, de la Rosa M, Salido M, Melero C, Rodríguez-Rivera M, Bougeon S, Collado R, Gimeno E, García-Serra R, Alonso S, Moro-García MA, García-Malo MD, Calvo X, Arenillas L, Ferrer A, Mantere T, Hoischen A, Schoumans J, Espinet B. Optical genome mapping: A promising new tool to assess genomic complexity in chronic lymphocytic leukemia (CLL). Cancers (Basel). 2022;**14**(14):3376. DOI: 10.3390/cancers14143376

[20] Levy B, Baughn LB, Akkari Y, Chartrand S, LaBarge B, Claxton D, Lennon PA, Cujar C, Kolhe R, Kroeger K, Pitel B, Sahajpal N, Sathanoori M, Vlad G, Zhang L, Fang M, Kanagal-Shamanna R, Broach JR. Optical genome mapping in acute myeloid leukemia: A multicenter evaluation. Blood Advances. 2023;**7**(7):1297–1307. DOI: 10.1182/bloodadvances.2022007583

[21] Neveling K, Mantere T, Vermeulen S, Oorsprong M, van Beek R, Kater-Baats E, Pauper M, van der Zande G, Smeets D, Weghuis DO, Stevens-Kroef MJPL, Hoischen A. Next-generation cytogenetics: Comprehensive assessment of 52 hematological malignancy genomes by optical genome mapping. American Journal of Human Genetics. 2021;**108**(8):1423–1435. DOI: 10.1016/j.ajhg.2021.06.001

[22] Ramos-Campoy S, Puiggros A, Kamaso J, Beà S, Bougeon S, Larráyoz MJ, Costa D, Parker H, Rigolin GM, Blanco ML, Collado R, Ancín I, Salgado R, Moro-García MA, Baumann T, Gimeno E, Moreno C, Salido M, Calvo X, Calasanz MJ, Cuneo A, Nguyen-Khac F, Oscier D, Haferlach C, Strefford JC, Schoumans J, Espinet B. TP53 abnormalities are underlying the poor outcome associated with chromothripsis in chronic lymphocytic leukemia patients with complex karyotype. Cancers (Basel). 2022;**14**(15):3715. DOI: 10.3390/cancers14153715

[23] Sahajpal NS, Mondal AK, Tvrdik T, Hauenstein J, Shi H, Deeb KK, Saxe D, Hastie AR, Chaubey A, Savage NM, Kota V, Kolhe R. Clinical validation and diagnostic utility of optical genome mapping for enhanced cytogenomic analysis of hematological neoplasms. Journal of Molecular Diagnostics. 2022;**24**(12):1279–1291. DOI: 10.1016/j.jmoldx.2022.09.009

[24] Smith AC, Neveling K, Kanagal-Shamanna R. Optical genome mapping for structural variation analysis in hematologic malignancies. American Journal of Hematology. 2022;**97**(7):975–982. DOI: 10.1002/ajh.26587

[25] Gupta A, Place M, Goldstein S, Sarkar D, Zhou S, Potamousis K, Kim J, Flanagan C, Li Y, Newton MA, Callander NS, Hematti P, Bresnick EH, Ma J, Asimakopoulos F, Schwartz DC. Single-molecule analysis reveals widespread structural variation in multiple myeloma. Proceedings of the National Academy of Sciences of the United States of America. 2015;**112**(25):7689–7694. DOI: 10.1073/pnas.1418577112

[26] Smith AC, Hoischen A, Raca G. Cytogenetics is a science, not a technique! Why optical genome mapping is so important to clinical genetic laboratories. Cancers (Basel). 2023;**15**(22):5470. DOI: 10.3390/cancers15225470

[27] Visconte V, Shetty S, Przychodzen B, Hirsch C, Bodo J, Maciejewski JP, Hsi ED, Rogers HJ. Clinicopathologic and molecular characterization of myeloid neoplasms with isolated t(6;9)(p23;q34). International Journal of Laboratory Hematology. 2017;**9**(4):409–417. DOI: 10.1111/ijlh.12641

[28] Slovak ML, Gundacker H, Bloomfield CD, Dewald G, Appelbaum FR, Larson RA, Tallman MS, Bennett JM, Stirewalt DL, Meshinchi S, Willman CL, Ravindranath Y, Alonzo TA, Carroll AJ, Raimondi SC, Heerema NA. A retrospective study of 69 patients with t(6;9)(p23;q34) AML emphasizes the need for a prospective, multicenter initiative for rare 'poor prognosis' myeloid malignancies. Leukemia. 2006;**20**(7):1295–1297. DOI: 10.1038/sj.leu.2404233

[29] Panagopoulos I, Gorunova L, Torkildsen S, Tjønnfjord GE, Micci F, Heim S. DEK-NUP214-fusion identified by RNA-sequencing of an acute myeloid leukemia with t(9;12)(q34;q15). Cancer Genomics & Proteomics. 2017;**14**(6):437–443. DOI: 10.21873/cgp.20053

[30] Smith AC, Maze D, Xia D, Capo-Chichi JM, King I, Sibai H. A t(6;14;9)(p22;q22;q34) three-way translocation: Description of a cytogenetically visible variant t(6;9) in acute myeloid leukemia. American Journal of Hematology. 2022;**97**(7):983–985. DOI: 10.1002/ajh.26534

[31] Qu S, Yan Y, Li C, Xu Z, Cai W, Qin T, Zhang P, Jia Y, Pan L, Gao Q, Li B, Liu J, Jiao M, Xiao Z. Case of cryptic TNIP1::PDGFRB rearrangement presenting with myelodysplastic syndrome achieved hematologic and cytogenetic remission with low-dose imatinib plus decitabine therapy. Leukemia Research Reports. 2023;**19**:100367. DOI: 10.1016/j.lrr.2023.100367

[32] Akkari Y, Baughn LB, Kim A, Karaca E, Raca G, Shao L, Mikhail FM. ACMG Laboratory Quality Assurance Committee. Section E6.1-6.6 of the American College of Medical Genetics and Genomics (ACMG) Technical Laboratory Standards: Cytogenomic studies of acquired chromosomal abnormalities in neoplastic blood, bone marrow, and lymph nodes. Genetics in Medicine. 2024;**26**(4):101054. DOI: 10.1016/j.gim.2023.101054

[33] WHO Classification of Haematolymphoid Tumour. 5th. who.int

[34] Xu X, Bryke C, Sukhanova M, Huxley E, Dash DP, Dixon-Mciver A, Fang M, Griepp PT, Hodge JC, Iqbal A, Jeffries S, Kanagal-Shamanna R, Quintero-Rivera F, Shetty S, Slovak ML, Yenamandra A, Lennon PA, Raca G. Assessing copy number abnormalities and copy-neutral loss-of-heterozygosity across the genome as best practice in diagnostic evaluation of acute myeloid leukemia: An evidence-based review from the cancer genomics consortium (CGC) myeloid neoplasms working group. Cancer Genetics. 2018;**228-229**:218–235. DOI: 10.1016/j.cancergen.2018.07.005

[35] Zhang X, Sjöblom T. Targeting loss of heterozygosity: A novel paradigm for cancer therapy. Pharmaceuticals (Basel). 2021;**14**(1):57. DOI: 10.3390/ph14010057

[36] Chauffaille MLLF, Zalcberg I, Barreto WG, Bendit I. Detection of somatic TP53 mutations and 17p deletions in patients with chronic lymphocytic leukemia: A review of the current methods. Hematology, Transfusion and Cell Therapy. 2020;**42**(3):261–268. DOI: 10.1016/j.htct.2020.05.005

[37] Fitzgibbon J, Smith LL, Raghavan M, Smith ML, Debernardi S, Skoulakis S, Lillington D, Lister TA, Young BD. Association between acquired uniparental disomy and homozygous gene mutation in acute myeloid leukemias. Cancer Research. 2005;**65**(20):9152–9154. DOI: 10.1158/0008-5472.CAN-05-2017

[38] National Comprehensive Cancer Network (NCCN). Clinical Practice Guidelines in Oncology (NCCN Guidelines®). NCCN.org: Myelodysplastic Syndromes Version 3; 2024

[39] Shah YB, Priore SF, Li Y, Tang CN, Nicholas P, Kurre P, Olson TS, Babushok DV. The predictive value of PNH clones, 6p CN-LOH, and clonal TCR gene rearrangement for aplastic anemia diagnosis. Blood Advances. 2021;**5**(16):3216–3226. DOI: 10.1182/bloodadvances.2021004201

[40] Katagiri T, Sato-Otsubo A, Kashiwase K, Morishima S, Sato Y, Mori Y, Kato M, Sanada M, Morishima Y, Hosokawa K, Sasaki Y, Ohtake S, Ogawa S, Nakao S, Japan Marrow Donor Program. Frequent loss of HLA alleles associated with copy number-neutral 6pLOH in acquired aplastic anemia. Blood. 2011;**118**(25):6601–6609. DOI: 10.1182/blood-2011-07-365189

[41] Ballesta-Alcaraz L, Bernal M, Vilchez JR, Palacios JA, Jiménez P, Garrido P, Gutiérrez-Bautista JF, Ruiz-Cabello F. Application of optical genome mapping for the diagnosis and risk stratification of myeloid and lymphoid malignancies. International Journal of Molecular Sciences. 2025;**26**(12):5763. DOI: 10.3390/ijms26125763

[42] Daneshbod Y, Kohan L, Taghadosi V, Weinberg OK, Arber DA. Prognostic significance of complex karyotypes in acute myeloid leukemia. Current Treatment Options in Oncology. 2019;**20**(2):15. DOI: 10.1007/s11864-019-0612-y

[43] Holland AJ, Cleveland DW. Chromoanagenesis and cancer: Mechanisms and consequences of localized, complex chromosomal rearrangements. Nature Medicine. 2012;**18**(11):1630–1638. DOI: 10.1038/nm.2988

[44] Guermouche H, Roynard P, Penther D, Daudignon A. Chromoanagenesis in multiple myeloma: A comprehensive overview. Methods in Molecular Biology. 2025;**2968**:343–360. DOI: 10.1007/978-1-0716-4750-9_20

[45] Ramos-Campoy S, Kamaso J, Puiggros A, Espinet B. Chromoanagenesis detection in chronic lymphocytic leukemia. Methods in Molecular Biology. 2025;**2968**:231–248. DOI: 10.1007/978-1-0716-4750-9_13

[46] Wei Q, Hu S, Loghavi S, Toruner GA, Ravandi-Kashani F, Tang Z, Li S, Xu J, Daver N, Medeiros LJ, Tang G. Chromoanagenesis is frequently associated with highly complex

karyotypes, extensive clonal heterogeneity, and treatment refractoriness in acute myeloid leukemia. American Journal of Hematology. 2025;**100**(3):417–426. DOI: 10.1002/ajh.27575

[47] Toruner GA, Hu S, Loghavi S, Ok CY, Tang Z, Wei Q, Kanagal-Shamanna R, Medeiros LJ, Tang G. Clinical utility of optical genome mapping as an additional tool in a standard cytogenetic workup in hematological malignancies. Cancers (Basel). 2025;**17**(9):1436. DOI: 10.3390/cancers17091436

[48] Smith AC, Tsui H, Usta S, Capo-Chichi JM. What the VAF? A guide to the interpretation of variant allele fraction, percent mosaicism, and copy number in cancer. Molecular Cytogenetics. 2025;**18**(1):13. DOI: 10.1186/s13039-025-00718-3

[49] Choi SM, Dewar R, Burke PW, Shao L. Partial tandem duplication of KMT2A (MLL) may predict a subset of myelodysplastic syndrome with unique characteristics and poor outcome. Haematologica. 2018;**103**(3):e131–e134. DOI: 10.3324/haematol.2017.185249

[50] Akkari YMN, Bruyere H, Hagelstrom RT, Kanagal-Shamanna R, Liu J, Luo M, Mikhail FM, Pitel BA, Raca G, Shago M, Shao L, Smith LR, Smolarek TA, Yenamandra A, Baughn LB. Evidence-based review of genomic aberrations in B-lymphoblastic leukemia/lymphoma: Report from the cancer genomics consortium working group for lymphoblastic leukemia. Cancer Genetics. 2020;**243**:52–72. DOI: 10.1016/j.cancergen.2020.03.001

[51] Yenamandra AK, Smith RB, Senaratne TN, Kang SL, Fink JM, Corboy G, Hodge CA, Lu X, Mathew S, Crocker S, Fang M. Evidence-based review of genomic aberrations in diffuse large B cell lymphoma, not otherwise specified (DLBCL, NOS): Report from the cancer genomics consortium lymphoma working group. Cancer Genetics. 2022;**268-269**:1–21. DOI: 10.1016/j.cancergen.2022.07.006

[52] Pugh TJ, Fink JM, Lu X, Mathew S, Murata-Collins J, Willem P, Fang M, Cancer Genomics Consortium Plasma Cell Disorders Working Group. Assessing genome-wide copy number aberrations and copy-neutral loss-of-heterozygosity as best practice: An evidence-based review from the cancer genomics consortium working group for plasma cell disorders. Cancer Genetics. 2018;**228-229**:184–196. DOI: 10.1016/j.cancergen.2018.07.002

[53] Geiersbach KB, Chen H, Emmadi R, Haskell GT, Lu X, Liu YJ, Swisshelm K. Current concepts in breast cancer genomics: An evidence based review by the CGC breast cancer working group. Cancer Genetics. 2020;**244**:11–20. DOI: 10.1016/j.cancergen.2020.02.002

[54] Neill SG, Hauenstein J, Li MM, Liu YJ, Luo M, Saxe DF, Ligon AH. Copy number assessment in the genomic analysis of CNS neoplasia: An evidence-based review from the cancer genomics consortium (CGC) working group on primary CNS tumors. Cancer Genetics. 2020;**243**:19–47. DOI: 10.1016/j.cancergen.2020.02.004

[55] Liu YJ, Houldsworth J, Emmadi R, Dyer L, Wolff DJ. Assessing genomic copy number alterations as best practice for renal cell neoplasia: An evidence-based review from the cancer genomics consortium workgroup. Cancer Genetics. 2020;**244**:40–54. DOI: 10.1016/j.cancergen.2020.04.004

Chapter 2

# Chronic Myelogenous Leukaemia in the Era of Molecular Therapy

*Ibrahim O. Ahmed, Kaladada I. Korubo,*
*Rahman A. Bolarinwa and Muheez A. Durosinmi*

## Abstract

Chronic myeloid leukaemia (CML) is aetiologically linked to a genetic abnormality called the Philadelphia chromosome (Ph), which results from a reciprocal translocation between the long arms of chromosomes 9 and 22, leading to a shortened chromosome 22. This abnormality produces the BCR::ABL1 oncoprotein with inherent tyrosine kinase activity. Over 90% of patients have both the Ph karyotype and the BCR::ABL1 fusion protein, while 5%–10% express only the fusion protein. Although the main cause of CML remains unknown, exposure to ionizing radiation has been suggested as a factor. The disease's incidence is approximately 1–2 per 100,000 annually worldwide, with a slight male predominance. Median onset ages are 30 to 40 years in low- and middle-income countries, compared to 60 years and older in high-income regions. CML progresses through three phases: chronic phase (CP), accelerated phase (AP) with 10%–19% blasts, and blast phase (BP) with over 20% blasts. The advent of tyrosine kinase inhibitors (TKIs) has greatly improved survival rates, prompting the WHO in 2022 to reclassify CML as a two-stage disease – CP and BP – removing the AP category from its classification of hematolymphoid tumours. Patients successfully treated with TKIs now have lifespans similar to age-matched healthy individuals, even in low-income countries where these drugs are accessible. The effectiveness of TKIs has significantly reduced the need for allogeneic stem cell transplantation (Allo-SCT) in CML treatment. Nevertheless, other medications such as hydroxyurea and cytarabine still play a role in managing certain cases.

**Keywords:** chronic myeloid leukaemia, Philadelphia chromosome, Imatinib, tyrosine kinase inhibitors, BCR::ABL1

## 1. Introduction

The classic chronic myeloid leukaemia (CML), a myeloproliferative neoplasm (MPN), is characterized as BCR::ABL1-positive or JAK2V617F-negative leukaemia. It differs clinically from the other three MPNs – polycythaemia vera, essential thrombocythaemia (ET), and idiopathic myelofibrosis – which show JAK2V617F and other mutations such as MPL and calreticulin (CALR) [1]. Mutations in the MPL and

CALR genes promote the development of MPNs. The W515L mutation in MPL activates the thrombopoietin receptor, leading to megakaryopoiesis and ET and primary myelofibrosis (PMF), while the CALR mutation induces PMF [2]. CML is distinct from other myeloproliferative disorders, such as chronic myelomonocytic leukaemia, chronic neutrophilic leukaemia (CNL), chronic eosinophilic leukaemia, chronic basophilic leukaemia, and juvenile myelomonocytic leukaemia, which are Ph-negative [3]. In humans, CML was the first cancer linked to a genetic abnormality – the Philadelphia (Ph) chromosome – formed by a reciprocal translocation between chromosomes 9 and 22, t(9;22)(q34;q11), present in over 95% of cases. This translocation relocates the Abl tyrosine kinase gene on chromosome 9 to the BCR gene on chromosome 22, creating the oncogenic fusion gene BCR::ABL1 with strong tyrosine kinase activity, promoting tumour growth [4]. A variant lacking the Ph chromosome and BCR::ABL1, known as Ph-negative or atypical CML (aCML), retains an intact chromosome 22 with the breakpoint at 9q34 and occurs in 2%–5% of cases. Historically, aCML was considered a myeloproliferative subtype of CML [5]. However, the 2008 and 2016 WHO classifications clarified that it is not a variant of CML or BCR::ABL1-positive diseases [6, 7]. Compared to CML, aCML is a rare and aggressive MPN, with no standard treatment, a poor prognosis, and low survival rates [5]. In 1845, Rudolf Virchow in Berlin and John Hughes Bennet in Edinburgh independently identified CML as a suppurative blood disorder marked by high white blood cell (WBC) count and splenomegaly [8, 9]. The BCR::ABL1 oncoprotein varies in size from 185/190 kDa to 230 kDa, depending on the breakpoint site in the BCR gene, but each fusion gene encodes the same part of the Abl tyrosine kinase. The BCR genes expressed in CML produce p210 kDa in 95%, p185/190 kDa in 1%, and p230 kDa in CNL [10].

CML primarily manifests as a triphasic clonal neoplasm, comprising the chronic phase (CP), the more aggressive accelerated phase (AP), and the terminal blastic phase (BP). The advent of imatinib and other TKI therapies has significantly enhanced survival rates for CML patients, leading the WHO to update its classification in 2022 by distinguishing CML into a biphasic clonal neoplasm – CP and BP – effectively removing AP from its categorization [11]. Patients effectively treated with TKIs now have lifespans comparable to their healthy, agematched counterparts [12]. Molecular diagnosis and ongoing monitoring are crucial for detecting mutations, evaluating treatment success, and identifying resistant clones. Achieving a major molecular response (MMR), marked by a 3-log reduction in BCR/ABL1 to ≤ 0.1%, is a key goal. Additionally, treatment-free remission (TFR) represents another major success achieved through TKI therapy [13].

## 2. Epidemiology and aetiology

Globally, CML accounts for approximately 15%–20% of all adult leukaemias, with an annual incidence of about 1–2 cases per 100,000 people [13]. The reported incidence in Africa is lower, at 0.4–1.0 per 100,000, which may result from underdiagnosis or underreporting rather than a true lower occurrence compared to Western countries [14]. Due to its chronic nature, CML comprises a larger share of adult leukaemia cases in Africa, sometimes being the most common type in certain countries, possibly linked to underdiagnosis of acute leukaemias. With advances in targeted therapies improving survival, CML's prevalence is rising. In the West, the median age at diagnosis is 55–60 years, while in low- and middle-income countries, it is lower, at 35–40 years, with some reports noting 25%–30% of cases diagnosed before age 30 [4]. The reasons for this age difference between Africa and the global average remain unclear. CML is uncommon in children. In Nigeria, the median age of patients on TKIs was 37 years (range 10–87), with a male-to-female ratio of 1.5:1 [15]. Biological and environmental risk factors include exposure to the Hiroshima and Nagasaki bombs, which showed peak incidence about six years after exposure [16], and benzene exposure [17]. Other potential but not confirmed risk factors are treatment with DNA topoisomerase inhibitors like etoposide [18] and smoking [19]. CML does not run in families; monozygotic twins and relatives are not at increased risk of developing the disease [18].

## 3. Pathogenesis

CML results from a spontaneous reciprocal translocation between chromosomes 9 and 22, creating the cytogenetic hallmark t(9;22)(q34;q11). This translocation fuses the Abelson proto-oncogene 1 (ABL1) on chromosome 9 with the breakpoint cluster region (BCR) gene on chromosome 22, transforming the latter into the Ph chromosome [1, 5]. The process leads to the formation of the oncogenic BCR::ABL1 fusion gene, which encodes a constitutively active tyrosine kinase, driving CML development. The BCR gene breakpoint varies, resulting in different fusion gene variants. The most common involves the major BCR region (M-BCR), producing the 210-kilodalton (kDa) (p210) fusion protein (BCR::ABL1 P210), primarily seen in typical CML (95%) and approximately one-third of Ph+ ALL (Ph+ acute lymphoblastic leukaemia [ALL]). About 97%–98% of CML cases express a chimeric mRNA with BCR exon 13 or 14 joined to ABL1 exon 2 (e13a2 and e14a2), forming specific fusion proteins[2]. Rarely, around 5% of patients develop signs and symptoms similar to CML, such as leukocytosis with a left shift, splenomegaly, and significant myeloid dysplasia, but test negative for both Ph and the BCR::ABL1 fusion gene. This aCML has a very poor prognosis [1, 5].

The frequencies of the transcript break points among the 230 Nigerian CML cases are as follows: the major (M-BCR) 210 kDa (p210 BCR::ABL1) involving exon 2 of ABL, e13a2, e14a2, and both e13a2 and e14a2 were 30 (13.0%), 114 (49.6%), and 82 (35.7%), respectively. The minor (190-kDa) in Ph+ ALL and micro (230-kDa) in CNL were rare, occurring at only 0.4% and 1.3%, respectively [20].

## 4. Clinical features

CML is a MPN that can be biphasic or triphasic. Its three stages include the indolent CP, the aggressive AP, and the terminal blastic phase. Clinical manifestations vary depending on the disease stage at diagnosis. Typically, 20%–50% of patients are asymptomatic and diagnosed via routine blood tests. Symptoms may include signs of hyperviscosity, such as headache, dizziness, blurred vision, tinnitus, low-grade fever, excessive sweating, and weight loss due to hypermetabolism. Some patients experience anaemia symptoms, like fatigue and weakness; thrombocytopenia signs, notably in the blastic stage, such as petechial and purpuric eruptions, and sometimes mucosal bleeding. Splenomegaly is frequently observed and may be associated with hepatomegaly. The emergence of palpable body masses, called chloromas, signals progression to the blastic phase [3, 10].

CML progresses through three main stages: the CP, AP, and blast crisis (BP). Although some reports describe a biphasic pattern where the disease moves directly from CP to BP without an intervening AP, patients can present in any of these stages. Nonetheless, most cases are diagnosed during the CP. The transition from CP to more advanced stages is not completely understood but is thought to be driven by genomic instability [13].

The CP is marked by leukocytosis levels between 20 and 200 $\times 10^9$ cells/L. Peripheral blood smears typically show a dominance of differentiating granulocytes, including myelocytes, metamyelocytes, and polymorphonuclear cells. Blast or promyelocyte percentages are usually below 10%, and there may be mild increases in basophils and eosinophils. Platelet counts are generally normal or increased, while anaemia is usually mild to moderate. Most patients are asymptomatic but might experience symptoms such as anaemia, fatigue, weight loss, and abdominal swelling or discomfort caused by splenomegaly. No additional cytogenetic clonal evolution is usually observed at this stage, aside from the presence of the Ph+/BCR::ABL1 fusion gene. Without treatment, the CP of CML lasts approximately two to seven years [3, 10, 13].

The AP is characterized by one or more of these features: 10%–19% blasts and promyelocytes in blood or bone marrow; over 20% basophils in peripheral blood; persistent thrombocytopenia (<100 $\times 10^9$ cells/L) not related to therapy, or ongoing thrombocytosis (>1,000 $\times 10^9$/L) unresponsive to treatment; increasing spleen size and rising WBC count that do not improve with therapy; megakaryocytic proliferation in large sheets and clusters with significant reticulin or collagen fibrosis; or evidence of clonal evolution. Patients in this stage often have symptoms but can also be asymptomatic. Besides features of CML-CP, they may experience systemic symptoms such as fever, weight loss, bone pain, and worsening anaemia or thrombocytopenia. Without treatment, AP usually advances to the blastic phase within one to two years [3].

The blastic phase is marked by the presence of one or more features: blast cells making up at least 20% in the peripheral blood or nucleated bone marrow cells; extramedullary blast growth, such as in soft tissue chloromas or lymphadenopathy; large areas or clusters of blasts seen in a bone marrow biopsy; or evidence of clonal evolution. It can be classified as myeloid BP (70%), lymphoid BP (20%), or undifferentiated BP (10%). The lymphoblastic phase is more common in younger patients [3]. Patients with BP may not show symptoms but often display signs of hypercatabolism, a high tumour burden, bone marrow failure (leading to anaemia, bleeding, and infections), and multiple organ failure. Rare symptoms like Sweet syndrome (acute febrile neutrophilic dermatosis), spontaneous spleen rupture, digital necrosis, or neurological issues from central nervous system involvement (around 30% of lymphoid blastic phase cases) have been reported. Without treatment, the blastic phase typically has a survival time of three to six months [3, 10, 13].

The recent World Health Organization (WHO) definition of CML stages divides disease progression into two phases: an AP with continuous or increasing splenomegaly and persistent or increasing leucocytosis. Blast cell count ranges from 10% to 19%, basophil count exceeds 20%, and platelet count exceeds 1,000 $\times 10^9$/L. AP is also characterized by the presence of additional chromosomal aberrations

*DOI: http://dx.doi.org/10.5772/intechopen.1014112*

| Year | Chronic phase (CP) | Accelerated phase (AP) | Blast phase (BP) |
|---|---|---|---|
| **2016** | Blasts (peripheral blood [PB] and bone marrow [BM]) < 10%. | Blasts (PB or BM) 10%–19%, PB basophils ≥ 20%, platelets < 100 or > 1,000 × $10^9$/L – unrelated or unresponsive to treatment. Splenomegaly unresponsive to treatment. Rising WCC unresponsive to treatment. ACA at diagnosis, including 3q26.2 rearrangements, + 8, i(17q), + 19, + Ph, complex karyotype. ACA emerging on treatment. | Blasts (PB or BM) ≥ 20% extramedullary blast proliferation. |
| **2022** | Blasts (PB and BM) < 20%. High-risk indicators at diagnosis; high ELTS score.<br>Blasts (PB and BM) 10%–19%. PB basophils ≥ 20%, ACA: 3q26.2 rearrangements, - 7, i(17q) and complex karyotype.<br>Clusters of small megakaryocytes with fibrosis. High-risk indicators.<br>On treatment: No CHR on first-line TKI; resistance to 2GTKI (unless due to a BCR::ABL1 mutation); development of ACA.<br>Compound mutations in BCR:: ABL1. | No longer exists. | Blasts (PB or BM) ≥ 20% extramedullary blast proliferation.<br>Bona fide lymphoblasts in PB or BM (even if < 10%). |

**Table 1.**
*WHO definitions of clinical phases of CML, 2016 and 2022. Source: From literature [7, 8].*

(trisomy 8, isochromosome 17q, trisomy 19) during treatment or at diagnosis, as well as the occurrence of two or more mutations (mainly T315I) during therapy. The blastic phase is characterized by 20% or more blasts in blood, bone marrow, and extramedullary sites, along with splenomegaly and genomic evolution (emergence of additional cytogenetic abnormalities) [10]. The clinical features are summarized in **Table 1** below.

**Diagnostic work-up:** The definitive test for diagnosing CML is identifying Ph+ [t (9;22)(q34;q11)] using conventional cytogenetics or fluorescence *in situ* hybridization (FISH), or detecting BCR::ABL1 transcripts via Q-PCR. While the diagnostic process for CML typically starts with a full blood count, peripheral blood film, and bone marrow examination, these are standard investigations for CML patients [3].

**(1) Full blood count/Peripheral blood film examination**

The total leukocyte count is typically high at diagnosis, usually over 20 × $10^9$/L, with at least half of the patients exceeding 100 × $10^9$/L. Cyclic fluctuations in leukocyte levels occur in 10%–20% of cases. Thrombocytosis is seen in 30%–50% of patients and can surpass 1,000 × $10^9$/L, though platelet counts may also be normal or low. Platelet aggregation issues are common. Anaemia, defined as hemoglobin below 10 g/dL, occurs in 20% of cases. The absolute lymphocyte count may be elevated (average around 15 × $10^9$/L) at diagnosis, reflecting a balanced increase in T-helper and T-suppressor cells, whereas B lymphocytes usually remain unchanged. The peripheral blood smear shows increased myeloid cells across all maturation stages, from blasts to mature neutrophils, with intermediate myelocytes and neutrophils being predominant during the CP. Basophilia and eosinophilia can also be present. The disease phase can be assessed by examining the peripheral blood smear [3, 10].

(2) **Bone marrow morphology**

Bone marrow aspiration or trephine biopsy is not essential for diagnosing CML, but it is generally carried out to evaluate marrow fibrosis, perform cytogenetic analysis on marrow cells, and rule out early transformation. Marrow aspirates usually reveal hypercellularity with a raised myeloid-to-erythroid ratio (10:1 to 30:1), mainly due to an abundance of granulocytes, including basophil and eosinophil precursors. Erythropoiesis tends to be decreased, while megakaryocytes may be normal or increased; however, they can be reduced in cases of blastic transformation. Pseudo-Gaucher cells, macrophages formed by increased cellular glucocerebroside from rapid cell turnover, may also be observed. The marrow trephine biopsy displays a complete loss of fat spaces with dense hypercellularity. The reticulin content might be normal or slightly elevated [13].

(3) **Conventional cytogenetics**

Conventional cytogenetics typically uses bone marrow or peripheral blood samples. It identifies the Ph + chromosome through G-banding, which is present in about 90% of CML cases. The sample is incubated at 37°C with RPMI 1640 culture medium containing L-glutamine for 24 hours. Colchicine is then added for one to two hours to arrest cells at metaphase. Growth factors are included to stimulate cell division. The process continues with cell fixation, slide preparation, and G-banding. In standard practice, only 20 metaphases are analysed, and roughly 5% of patients may have an undetectable Ph chromosome. Conventional cytogenetics can also be used to detect the presence of other cytogenetic abnormalities associated with clonal evolution in CML, such as the loss of chromosome Y and trisomies +8 and +19 [21].

(4) **Fluorescent *in situ* hybridization**

FISH involves using specific DNA probes to detect 5′-BCR and 3′-ABL1 gene sequences on the Ph+ chromosome. The 5′-BCR probe is directly labeled with a Spectrum Green fluorophore, while the 3′-ABL1 probe is labeled with a Spectrum Orange fluorophore. When both probes hybridize, they produce an overlapping yellow fusion signal, indicating the BCR::ABL1 fusion gene. The close proximity of BCR and ABL1 signals identifies CML cells. FISH allows for the detection and quantification of the BCR::ABL1 oncogene in interphase or metaphase cells from peripheral blood samples. Typically, up to 200 nuclei are screened, increasing sensitivity and specificity compared to traditional cytogenetics, though there is a false-positive rate of 1% to 10%. FISH can also assess minimal residual disease (MRD) and detect unusual variants of the BCR::ABL1 gene rearrangement that RT-PCR primers may miss, including masked Ph+ chromosomes on chromosome 9 [21].

(5) **Quantitative reverse transcriptase polymerase chain reaction**
Reverse transcriptase quantitative polymerase chain reaction (RT-qPCR) is a molecular technique that measures BCR::ABL1 transcript levels in blood samples to evaluate the molecular response. It can detect one BCR::ABL1 transcript among $10^5$ normal cells and is the most sensitive and specific test available, making it ideal for assessing MRD in CML patients. This molecular response test can predict long-term outcomes such as overall survival (OS) and progression-free survival (PFS). Retrospective studies show that patients with stable MMR have higher OS and PFS compared to those who never reach MMR. In the IRIS trial, patients who achieved MMR by 18 months did not progress to advanced disease and had a 7-year event-free survival rate of 7%. Consequently, routine monitoring with RT-qPCR is an effective predictor of survival and is used to track treatment response at the molecular level in CML patients on TKIs or after allogeneic stem cell transplantation (Allo-SCT). It also allows early detection of clonal evolution and facilitates DNA sequencing for mutational analysis [22].

## 5. Treatment

The treatment of CML must be comprehensive and, like any other malignancy, should include counselling, supportive care, and definitive therapies.

## 6. Counselling

Counselling is crucial for patients who are newly diagnosed with CML and those receiving treatment. It is important to discuss key aspects with both the patient and their relatives. Counselling enhances understanding of the disease, available treatments, and possible outcomes, which can lead to improved adherence to therapy and follow-up appointments. Patients and their families should be educated about CML using simple and relatable language to ensure clear understanding. It is essential to explain that CML is a blood cancer that is neither inherited nor contagious. It should also be communicated that CML is a chronic, non-communicable disease manageable with TKIs, and that continuing treatment is vital even if symptoms improve. Patients should be advised not to stop therapy without consulting their healthcare providers [23].

## 7. Supportive care

Patients with CML require supportive therapies ranging from antibiotics to blood products, such as red cell and platelet transfusions, especially during the disease's blastic phase. Routine prophylactic antibiotics are not standard; however, CML patients face a high infection risk due to immunosuppression caused by neutropenia, hypogammaglobulinaemia, and impaired cellular function. Febrile neutropenia can occur during blastic transformation due to bone marrow suppression. It should be treated as an emergency, ideally with broad-spectrum antimicrobials guided by local culture and sensitivity data. Patients in the CP may have mildly elevated serum uric acid levels, though they are often normal. The rapid cell turnover increases the risk of tumour lysis syndrome, so serial assessments of uric acid and kidney function are recommended. Preventive measures include prophylaxis with xanthine oxidase inhibitors like allopurinol, along with IV fluids and electrolyte support, particularly in patients with markedly high WBC counts. Allopurinol should be stopped when the WBC count drops below $20 \times 10^9$/L. Rasburicase, an enzyme that converts uric acid to allantoin, is highly effective for managing hyperuricemia [3, 12].

## 8. Cytoreductive therapy

Cytoreductive therapy uses drugs like hydroxyurea and busulphan to reduce high WBC and, sometimes, platelet counts quickly. This approach is often vital in hyperleukocytosis cases to prevent or treat hyperviscosity syndrome. Although it is not a definitive solution, it provides rapid relief and helps prevent hyperviscosity complications like deafness and dizziness. Hydroxyurea, which inhibits ribonucleotide reductase and targets more mature myeloid progenitors in the proliferative cycle, is frequently used and should be stopped once the WBC count falls below $20 \times 10^9$/L. In emergencies, leukapheresis or plasmapheresis may be performed for urgent cytoreduction [3].

## 9. Prognostic scores in CML

For CML, the aim of TKI therapy is to attain and maintain remission, which can enable TFR. To predict disease outcomes and inform treatment choices, considering prognostic factors is crucial. This is why risk stratification at diagnosis, before starting TKI therapy, is recommended. Several validated risk scores are used for CML, including the Sokal score, the Hasford (Euro) score, the European Treatment and Outcome Study (EUTOS) score, and the EUTOS long-term survival score (ELTS). Although the Sokal score was developed prior to the availability of imatinib, it remains relevant today for predicting PFS and cytogenetic response in CML patients. The Hasford score, also called the Euro score, was created by Hasford and colleagues and requires parameters such as age, spleen size, blast count, platelet count, peripheral basophil percentage, and eosinophil counts. The EUTOS score, introduced in 2011, is a more recent score that predicts complete cytogenetic response and PFS in patients treated with imatinib. It is calculated using the formula: (7 × basophil [%]) + (4 × spleen [cm]). Patients are categorized into low-risk (score under 87) and high-risk (score of 87 or higher) groups, as per EUTOS. The ELTS score was developed based on data from 2,205 adult patients with Ph chromosome-positive and/or BCR-ABL1-positive chronic-phase CML, including transcript types e13a2 and/or e14a2, who received imatinib within six months of diagnosis. All these scoring systems have been validated for patients on TKI therapy, but no single score has been proven superior or more user-friendly. Moreover, there is no consistent

| SOKAL [24] | EURO [25] | EUTOS [26] | ELTS [27] |
|---|---|---|---|
| Low risk: < 0.8 | Low risk: ≤ 780 | Low risk: ≤ 87 | < 1.5680 |
| Intermediate risk: 0.8–1.2 | Intermediate risk: 781–1,480 | None | 1.5680–2.2185 |
| High risk: > 1.2 | High risk: ≥ 1,480 | High risk: > 87 | >2.2185 |
| Exp 0.01169 (age in years -43.4) + 0.0345 × (spleen size -7.51) + 0.188 × ([platelet count ÷ 700]$^2$-0.563) +0.0887 × (blast cells-210) | 0.666 when age ≥ 50 years + (0.042 × spleen) + 1.0956 when platelet count > 1,500 × $10^9$L + (0.0584 × blast cells) + 0.20399 when basophils > 3% + (0.0413 × eosinophils) × 100 | Spleen × 4 + basophils × 7 | 0.0025 × (age/10)$^3$ + 0.0615 × spleen size + 0.1052 × blast percentage + 0.4104 × (platelet count/1,000)-0.5. |

**Table 2.**
*The interpretations of the prognostic scores in CML.*

evidence that intermediate-risk patients behave differently from low-risk ones. Therefore, patients are generally categorized into low- (including intermediate) and high-risk groups regardless of the scoring system, and these tools are available online for assessment. **Table 2** summarizes the interpretations of these scores [24–27].

## 10. Molecular therapy with TKI

The development of BCR::ABL1-targeted therapy with imatinib revolutionized CML treatment, turning a previously fatal disease into a manageable, chronic condition. Since its discovery, it has been shown to induce lasting remission and extend survival, with notable improvements over drugs like busulphan, hydroxyurea, and IFNα [28]. In Nigeria, since 2003, imatinib (Gleevec®) has been provided free to CML patients through the GIPAP program, now known as the Max Solution (MAS), led by Novartis and the Max Foundation. A preliminary report indicates durable remission with Gleevec in Nigerian patients, with OS rates of 95%, 90%, and 75% at one, two, and five years, respectively [15]. Evidence now suggests that CML patients' life expectancy is approaching that of the general population [12]. Imatinib mesylate, a first-generation tyrosine kinase inhibitor (TKI), remains the main treatment for CML. Second-generation TKIs – dasatinib, bosutinib, and nilotinib – are typically reserved for cases resistant or intolerant to imatinib. Resistance to imatinib can occur through BCR::ABL1-dependent mechanisms involving kinase domain mutations or via BCR::ABL1-independent mechanisms caused by factors such as pharmacokinetic variability, non-adherence, incorrect drug combinations, or cytogenetic abnormalities [29]. The recently approved third-generation agent (3GN), ponatinib, is a multitargeted TKI designed for patients with the T315I mutation or CML resistant to all other TKIs [30].

Furthermore, new targeted therapies for BCR::ABL1 are being developed, mainly for third-line treatment and patients with the T315I mutation. Vodobatinib is a novel drug tested in CML patients resistant or intolerant to at least three TKIs or with comorbidities that restrict TKI use. It has shown *in vitro* effectiveness against most BCR::ABL1 mutations and is under investigation as a potential new treatment for CML. Olverembatinib, a third-generation TKI, demonstrated efficacy in a phase I study, especially for patients with the T315I mutation or those refractory or intolerant to other TKIs. PF-114, a fourth-generation TKI structurally similar to ponatinib, targets.

BCR::ABL1 mutations at nanomolar concentrations. It is effective in patients who have failed two or more TKIs or carry the T315I mutation [29]. Another promising targeted therapy is asciminib (ABL001), the first allosteric BCR::ABL1 inhibitor, which binds to the myristoylated site of the ABL protein and allosterically inhibits BCR::ABL1 kinase activity by stabilizing its inactive form. It received FDA accelerated approval in 2021 and has shown good efficacy in patients who have failed two or more TKIs or have the T315I mutation [31].

## 11. Definition of response to therapy

The primary treatment guidelines for monitoring CML patients on imatinib from organizations like National Comprehensive Cancer Network (NCCN), European Leukaemia Network (ELN), and European Society for Medical Oncology (ESMO) recommend using tests such as full blood count/peripheral blood film, conventional cytogenetics or FISH, and quantitative RT-PCR BCR::ABL1 mRNA transcript to assess haematologic, cytogenetic, and molecular responses, respectively [32–34]. The different terms used to describe responses include:

- **Complete haematologic response (CHR)** is defined by a WBC count less than $10 \times 10^9$/L with a normal differential, a platelet count below $450 \times 10^9$/L, no circulating immature cells in peripheral blood, and the resolution of all signs and symptoms of the disease, including palpable splenomegaly.

- **Partial haematologic response (PHR)** indicates the presence of immature blood cells in the peripheral blood, a platelet count less than 50% of the pre-treatment level but greater than $450 \times 10^9$/L, and/or persistent splenomegaly (but less than 50% of the pre-treatment size).

- **Complete cytogenetic response (CCyR);** when there are no Ph+ metaphases (0 Ph+ out of 20 metaphases) in the bone marrow.

- **Major cytogenetic response (MCyR)** occurs when there are 0%–35% Ph+ metaphases (0 to 7 Ph+ out of 20 metaphases) in the bone marrow.

- **Minor cytogenetic response (minor CyR);** when there are > 35% Ph+ metaphases (8–19 Ph+ out of 20 metaphases) in the bone marrow.

- **MMR;** when there is a ≥ 3-log reduction of BCR::ABL mRNA or a BCR::ABL/ABL ratio of < 0.1% on the International Scale.

- **Deep molecular response (DMR);** when there is ≥ 4.5-log reduction of BCR::ABL mRNA or a BCR::ABL/ABL ratio of < 0.01% on the International Scale.

- **Complete molecular response (CMR);** when BCR::ABL mRNA is undetectable by RT-qPCR or the BCR::ABL/ABL ratio is < 0.001% on the International Scale.

## 12. TFR in CML

Currently, the management of CML is shifting from continuous TKI therapy toward aiming for TKI discontinuation. TFR refers to a period of sustained molecular remission in CML patients after stopping TKI therapy. While stopping treatment after reaching control targets is uncommon in other chronic conditions like diabetes or hypertension, it is a significant focus of research in CML. Factors such as therapy costs, long-term TKI side effects, reduced quality of life (QOL), and anxiety about long-term cancer treatment drive ongoing research into TKI discontinuation [35]. Although eligibility criteria vary between studies, the NCCN guideline states TKI cessation may be considered when: patients are 18 or older, in the CP of CML without prior accelerated or blast phase (BP), have a measurable BCR::ABL1 transcript, have received at least three years of TKI therapy with a minimum of two years of stable MR 4.0, and have access to reliable Q-PCR monitoring during follow-up. For instance, in December 2017, the FDA updated its label for nilotinib to include indications for stopping therapy in patients who have been on nilotinib for at least three years, achieved a sustained MR 4.0 (BCR::ABL1 IS ≤ 0.01%) for one year before discontinuation, and reached MR 4.5 (BCR::ABL1 IS ≤ 0.0032%) before stopping. Patients must also have the major BCR::ABL1 transcript (e13a2/b2a2 or e14a2/b3a2). Ph+ CML-CP patients resistant or intolerant to imatinib who achieve sustained MR 4.0 while on nilotinib may qualify for TFR if they meet earlier criteria and have no history of accelerated or BP or previous failed TFR attempts [36]. After meeting these criteria, a thorough discussion of the benefits and risks of TKI cessation with the patient is essential before attempting TFR. Patient willingness is crucial; a survey by Goldberg et al. [37] of 210 CML patients at a single centre revealed that only 42% were willing to try TKI discontinuation, 34% preferred to continue therapy, and 25% were undecided. Reasons for discontinuation included side effects (40%), costs (30%), and inconvenience (26%). Reasons against discontinuation included fear of disease recurrence (58%) and absence of current toxicities (17%) [37]. During TFR, monthly Q-PCR monitoring is recommended in the first year, then every six weeks in the second year, and every 12 weeks thereafter [36]. Some patients experienced musculoskeletal and joint pain after stopping imatinib therapy [38]. This was specifically analysed in a subset of the EURO-SKI trial, where 15 out of 50 patients reported such symptoms [39]. The pain affected various body parts, including the shoulder, hip, and extremities, sometimes resembling polymyalgia rheumatica. Most cases were mild and managed with over-thecounter medications like paracetamol or nonsteroidal anti-inflammatory drugs (NSAIDs), although some patients had more severe symptoms that disrupted daily life and required steroid treatment. Over time, these symptoms generally resolved. The exact mechanisms remain unclear, but prolonged c-Kit inhibition by TKI, especially imatinib, may explain this syndrome. Long-term blocking of c-Kit has also been linked to skin and hair hypopigmentation observed with imatinib. Additionally, nilotinib has been used in a proof-of-concept study to treat spondyloarthritis, suggesting that mast cells might be the target cells involved in this syndrome. Ongoing research aims to clarify the potential connection [38].

## 13. Management of suboptimal response and treatment failure

Patients who are resistant or are becoming resistant to imatinib are at risk of disease progression. If a patient only achieves a suboptimal response or fails to respond to imatinib, mutation testing is recommended by ELN and NCCN before switching to another TKI or therapy. Early dose escalation of imatinib may overcome resistance. Studies show that increasing the dose to 600–800 mg daily helped some CML-CP patients with initial cytogenetic resistance achieve various levels of CHR and cytogenetic response. Dose escalation was also effective in patients on 300–400 mg/day with initial haematologic or cytogenetic resistance, with 65% and 56% achieving CHR and MCyR after dose increases to 600 or 800 mg. A trial found that starting at 600 mg resulted in higher response rates (55% MMR at 12 months and 77% at 24 months) than starting below 600 mg (32% and 77%, respectively). For patients with haematologic intolerance, increasing the dose is not appropriate and may not be feasible, necessitating a switch of therapy. Second-line TKIs like nilotinib, dasatinib, or bosutinib are recommended for patients with resistance or intolerance, or who do not reach treatment milestones with imatinib. The choice depends on safety, tolerability, comorbidities, mutation status, drug availability, cost, and clinician experience. Ponatinib, a third-generation TKI, is suitable for T315I mutation or resistance to second-line TKIs. Asciminib, which binds to ABL myristoyl pockets to inhibit ABL1 kinase, is approved for adults with resistant or intolerant chronic-phase CML after two or more TKIs, or with the T315I mutation. Omacetaxine or allogeneic stem cell transplant (SCT) are options for patients resistant or intolerant to imatinib and other TKIs [32–34].

## 14. TKI and fertility

Since TKI use has been linked to improved OS and QOL for CML patients, concerns about their impact on fertility have increased. Emerging evidence indicates that TKIs may impair fertility by blocking cKIT and platelet-derived growth factor receptor alpha (PDGFR-α), which are targeted by imatinib and other TKIs. c-KIT is present on human ovaries, and PDGFR-α is found on ovarian follicles. As a result, TKIs can interfere with primary follicle development, decreasing the overall follicle count by inhibiting these receptors [40]. Studies have shown that imatinib and other TKIs can impair oogenesis and follicular development [41]. However, there are reports of successful pregnancies and childbirth among women taking imatinib. Despite these findings, it is advisable to plan or delay pregnancy until the patient is in remission. Some patients have effectively used nonhormonal contraception or abstinence. In cases of unplanned pregnancy, it is recommended to temporarily stop TKIs during the first trimester and replace them with less teratogenic options like interferon alpha [42–44].

| | Guidelines<br>Response | ELN [32] | NCCN [33] | ESMO [34] | Remarks |
|---|---|---|---|---|---|
| Optimal response | Three months: CHR or Ph+ ≤ 35%, and/or BCR::ABL1 ≤ 10%.<br>Six months: Ph+ 0%, and/or BCR::ABL1 < 1%.<br>12 months: BCR::ABL1 ≤ 0.1%.<br>Any time: BCR::ABL1 ≤ 0.1%. | Three months: CHR or BCR::ABL1 ≤ 10% or (PCyR).<br>Six months: BCR::ABL1 ≤ 10% or ≥ PCyR.<br>12 months: CCyR) (if neither CCyR nor [MMR] has previously been achieved).<br>18 months: CCyR (if not in MMR and lacking CCyR at 12 months).<br>Any time: Stable or improving MMR. | Three months: 1+ CHR or ≤95%, or BCR-ABL1 < 10%.<br>< Six months: Ph + 0%, BCR::ABL1 1%.<br>< 12 months: BCR::ABL1 0.1%.<br><18 months: BCR::ABL1 0.01%. | | Optimal response means that the treatment should be continued because the response predicts an excellent outcome and an almost normal survival length. |
| Suboptimal response | Three months: Less than CHR or BCR::ABL1 > 10% and/or Ph+ 36%–95%.<br>Six months: BCR::ABL1 1-10% and/or Ph+ 1%–35% (PCyR).<br>12 months: BCR::ABL1 0.1%–1%. | Three months: Less than CHR or BCR::ABL1 > 10% or Ph+ 36%–95%.<br>Six months: BCR::ABL1 1–10% or Ph + 1–35% (PCyR).<br>12 months: BCR::ABL1 0.1%–1%. | Three months: Less than CHR or Ph+ 36%–95% and/or BCR::ABL > 10%.<br>Six months: Ph+ 1%–65% BCR::ABL 1%–10%.<br>12 months: BCR::ABL1 0.1%–1%.<br>>18 months: BCR::ABL1 0.1%–1%. | | Sub-optimal defines an intermediate category of response: This is the 'warning' category, and these patients require more frequent monitoring because continued benefit may occur from the current treatment or they may be possible consideration of change of treatment strategy due to an increased risk of failure. |

| | Guidelines Response | ELN [32] | NCCN [33] | ESMO [34] | Remarks |
|---|---|---|---|---|---|
| Treatment failure | Three months: Non-CHR and/or Ph+ > 95%.<br>Six months: BCR::ABL1 > 10% and/or Ph + > 35% (<PCyR).<br>12 months: BCR::ABL1 > 1% and/or Ph + ≥ 1%.<br>Any time: Loss of CHR, loss of CCyR, confirmed loss of MMR Mutations CCA/Ph+ | Three months: Non-CHR and/or Ph+ > 95%.<br>Six months: BCR::ABL1 > 10% and/or Ph + > 35% (<PCyR).<br>12 months: BCR::ABL1 > 1% and/or Ph+ ≥ 1%.<br>Any time: Loss of CHR, loss of CCyR, confirmed loss of MMR. | Three months: Non-CHR Ph+ > 95%.<br>Six months: Ph+ > 35% BCR::ABL1 > 10%.<br>12 months: Ph ≥ 1%.<br>Any time: Relapse or loss of MMR. | | Failed response to treatment indicates that the treatment should be changed because the response suggests that the patient is at a significant risk of disease progression and death. |

*Key: CHR: complete haematologic remission; Ph⁺: Philadelphia chromosome positive; PCyR: partial cytogenetic response; MMR: major molecular remission; CCR: complete cytogenetic remission.*

**Table 3.**
*The European Leukaemia Network (ELN), the National Comprehensive Cancer Network (NCCN), and the European Society for Medical Oncology (ESMO) definitions of treatment response.*

## 15. Treatment monitoring

Monitoring patients' response to imatinib or other TKIs is crucial because it guides clinical judgment and appropriate treatment. The guidelines generally classify patients into three groups: good responders (optimal response), poor responders (failed response or treatment failure), and the intermediate group (suboptimal response). These categories are based on the extent of haematologic, cytogenetic, and molecular response. **Table 3** summarizes the ELN, NCCN, and ESMO definitions of treatment response (optimal response, suboptimal response, and treatment failure) and the guidelines for monitoring response to imatinib in CML patients [32–34].

## 16. Stem cell transplantation

The NCCN guidelines recommend allogeneic SCT for patients who do not achieve certain treatment milestones with Tkis – such as a CHR within 3 months, partial CyR at 6 months, or CCyR within 12 months – or who are in the accelerated or BPs of the disease. Allogeneic SCT should also be considered for transplant-eligible patients who fail second- or third-line TKI therapy, and it is the preferred option for those showing clonal progression. While allogeneic SCT offers excellent long-term event-free survival rates of 40% to 80%, the one-year mortality can vary from 5% to 50%, influenced by factors such as age, stem cell source (related versus unrelated donor), mismatch degree, cytomegalovirus status, and prophylactic measures for infections and GVHD. The phase of the disease at SCT also impacts outcomes: relapse rates during transplantation in the CP are 5% to 20%, whereas in the accelerated or BPs, relapse may reach 30% to 60%. Relapse post-SCT can be managed with donor lymphocyte infusion (DLI), interferon therapy, or additional transplantation, although each has limitations. DLI can achieve CMRs (eliminating the BCR::ABL1 oncoprotein) in 60% to 70% of CP CML cases, but it may also lead to GVHD, myelosuppression, and potentially death.

The role of BCR::ABL1 testing after allogeneic SCT in predicting overall outcomes is significant. A positive QPCR result for BCR::ABL1 within 6 to 12 months post-transplant indicates a high relapse risk, whereas a positive result at much later times suggests a lower risk. Consequently, early detection of BCR::ABL1 transcripts posttransplant can help identify patients who may benefit from alternative treatments before a full relapse develops [45–47].

## Author details

Ibrahim O. Ahmed[1,2], Kaladada I. Korubo[3], Rahman A. Bolarinwa[1,2] and Muheez A. Durosinmi[4]*

1 Department of Haematology and Blood Transfusion, Obafemi Awolowo University Teaching Hospitals Complex, Ile-Ife, Nigeria

2 Department of Haematology and Immunology, Faculty of Basic Clinical Sciences, College of Health Sciences, Obafemi Awolowo University, Ile-Ife, Nigeria

3 Department of Haematology and Blood Transfusion, Faculty of Basic Clinical Sciences, College of Medical Sciences, Rivers State University, Port Harcourt, Nigeria

4 Department of Haematology, Faculty of Basic Medical Sciences, College of Health Sciences, Osun State University, Osogbo, Nigeria

*Address all correspondence to: mdurosin@gmail.com

## References

[1] Nowell PC, Hungerford DA. A minute chromosome in human granulocytic leukaemia. Science. 1960;**142**:1497

[2] Bench AJ, White HE, Foroni L, Godfrey AL, Gerrard G, Akiki S, Awan A, Carter I, Goday-Fernandez A, Langabeer SE, Clench T.Molecular diagnosis of the myeloproliferative neoplasms: UK guidelines for the detection of JAK 2 V 617 F and other relevant mutations. British Journal of Haematology. 2013;**60** (1):25–34

[3] Hoffbrand AV, Higgs DR, Keeling DM, AB M. Postgraduate Haematology. United Kingdom: John Wiley & Sons; 2016. 419–437 P

[4] Mendizabal AM, Younes N, Levine PH. Geographic and income variations in age at diagnosis and incidence of chronic myeloid leukemia. International Journal of Hematology. 2016;**103**(1):70–78

[5] L.C S, Mascarenhas J. Current and evolving understanding of atypical chronic myeloid leukaemia. Blood Reviews. 2019;**33**:74–81

[6] Vardiman JW, Adea TJ. The 2008 revision of the WHO classification of myeloid neoplasms and acute leukemia: Rationale and important changes. Blood. 2008;**114**(5):937–952

[7] Arber DA, Orazi A, Hasserjian R, Borowitz MJ, Le Beau MM, Bloomfield CD, et al. The 2016 revision of the World Health Organization classification of myeloid neoplasms and acute leukemia. Blood 2016;**127**:2391–2406

[8] Xiao W, Nardi V, Stein E, Hasserjian RP. A practical approach on the classifications of myeloid neoplasms and acute leukemia: WHO and ICC. Journal of Hematology & Oncology. 2024;**17**(1):1–16

[9] Virchow R. [Observation of increased white blood cells and initial use of the term 'leukämie']. [German]. 1845

[10] Hochhaus A, Saussele S, Rosti G, Mahon F-X, Janssen JJWM, H HH, et al. Chronic myeloid leukaemia: ESMO clinical practice guidelines for diagnosis, treatment and follow-up. Annals of Oncology. 2017;**28**:41–51

[11] Khoury JD, Solary E, Abla O, et al. The 5th edition of the World Health Organization classification of haematolymphoid tumours: Myeloid and histiocytic/dendritic neoplasms. Leukemia 2022;**36**:1703–1719

[12] Brower H, Bjorkholm M, Dickman PW, Hoglund M, Lambert PC, Andersson TM. Life expectancy of patients with chronic myeloid leukaemia approaches the life expectancy of the general population. Journal of Clinical Oncology. 2016;**34**:2851–2857

[13] Jabbour E, Kantarjian H. Chronic myeloid leukemia: 2025 update on diagnosis, therapy, and monitoring. American Journal of Hematology. 2024;**99**(11):2191–2212

[14] Obeagu EI, Omar DE, Bunu UO, Obeagu GU, Alum EU, Ugwu OP. Leukaemia burden in Africa. International Journal of Current Research in Biology and Medicine. 2023;**1**:17–22

[15] Oyekunle AA, Durosinmi MA, Bolarinwa RA, et al. Chronic myeloid leukemia in Nigerian patients: Anemia is an independent predictor of overall survival. Clinical Medicine Insights: Blood Disorders 2016;**20**:9–13

[16] Corso A, Lazzarino M, Morra E, Merante S, Astori C, Bernasconi P, Boni M, Bernasconi C. Chronic myelogenous leukemia and exposure to ionizing radiation–A retrospective study of 443 patients. Annals of Hematology. 1995;**70**(2):79–82

[17] Vlaanderen J, Lan Q, Kromhout H, Rothman N, Vermeulen R. Occupational benzene exposure and the risk of chronic myeloid leukemia: A meta-analysis of cohort studies incorporating study quality dimensions. American Journal of Industrial Medicine. 2012;**55** (9):779–785

[18] Pedersen-Bjergaard J, Brøndum-Nielsen K, Karle H, Johansson B. Chemotherapy-related – late occurring–Philadelphia chromosome in AML, ALL and CML. Similar events related to treatment with DNA topoisomerase II inhibitors? Leukemia. 1997;**11** (9):1571–1574

[19] Musselman JR, Blair CK, Cerhan JR, et al. Risk of adult acute and chronic myeloid leukemia with cigarette smoking and cessation. Cancer Epidemiology 2013;**37**:410–416

[20] Owojuyigbe TO, Durosinmi MA, Bolarinwa RAA, et al. Distribution of BCR-ABL1 transcript variants in Nigerians with chronic myeloid leukemia. Indian Journal of Hematology and Blood Transfusion 2020;**36**:646–651

[21] Altıntaş N, Aşçı M, Sarıcayılmaz Ö, Miskioğlu M, Kızıldağ S. Detection of Philadelphia chromosome and BCR-ABL fusion gene in patients with chronic myeloid leukemia by cytogenetic analysis and RT-PCR technique. Journal of Advanced Research in Health Sciences. 2021;**4** (2):1–6

[22] Kumar S, Gupta VK, Bharti A, Meena LP, Gupta V, Shukla J. A study to determine the clinical, hematological, cytogenetic, and molecular profile in CML patient in and around Eastern UP, India. Journal of Family Medicine and Primary Care. 2019;**8**(7):2450–2455

[23] Moon JH, Sohn SK, Kim SN, Park SY, Yoon SS, Kim IH, Kim HJ, Kim YK, Min YH, Cheong JW, Kim JS. Patient counseling program to improve the compliance to imatinib in chronic myeloid leukemia patients. Medical Oncology. 2012;**29**(2):1179–1185

[24] Sokal JE, Cox EB, Bacarrani M, Tura S, Gomez GA, Robertson JE. Prognostic indication in 'good-risk' chronic granulocytic leukaemia. Blood. 1984;**63**(4):789–799

[25] Hasford J, Pfirrmann M, Hehlmann R, Allan NC, Baccarani M, Kluin-Nelemans JC, et al. A new prognostic score for survival of patients with chronic myeloid leukaemia treated with interferon alfa. Journal of the National Cancer Institute. 1998;**90**:850–858

[26] Hasford J, Baccarani M, Hoffmann V, Guilhot J, Saussele S, Rosti G, et al. Predicting complete cytogenetic response and subsequent progression-free survival in 2060 patients with CML on imatinib treatment: The EUTOS score. Blood 2011;**118**:686–692

[27] Geelen IG, Sandin F, Thielen N, Janssen JJ, Hoogendoorn M, Visser O,

Cornelissen JJ, Hoglund M, Westerweel PE. Validation of the EUTOS long-term survival score in a recent independent cohort of "real world" CML patients. Leukemia. 2018;**32**(10):2299–2303

[28] Deininger M, Buchdunger E, Druker BJ. The development of imatinib as a therapeutic agent for chronic myeloid leukemia. Blood. 2005;**105**(7):2640–2653

[29] Tina Shih Y, Cortes JE, Kantarjian HM. Treatment value of second-generation BCR-ABL1 tyrosine kinase inhibitors compared with imatinib to achieve treatment free remission in patients with chronic myeloid leukaemia: A modelling study. The Lancet Hematology. 2019;**6**(8):e398–e408

[30] Malik S, Hassan S, Emre Eskazan A. Novel BCR-ABL1 tyrosine kinase inhibitors in the treatment of chronic myeloid leukaemia. Expert Review of Hematology. 2021;**14**(11):975–978

[31] Hochhaus A, Wang J, Kim DW, Kim DD, Mayer J, Goh YT, le Coutre P, Takahashi N, Kim I, Etienne G, Andorsky D. Asciminib in newly diagnosed chronic myeloid leukemia. New England Journal of Medicine. 2024;**391**(10):885–898

[32] Apperley JF, Milojkovic D, Cross NC, Hjorth-Hansen H, Hochhaus A, Kantarjian H, Lipton JH, Malhotra H, Niederwieser D, Radich J, Rousselot P. European LeukemiaNet recommendations for the management of chronic myeloid leukemia: Chronic myeloid leukemia. Leukemia. 2025;**2025**(11):1–7

[33] Jabbour E, Kantarjian H. Chronic myeloid leukemia: A review. Jama. 2025;**333**(18):1618–1629

[34] Eichhorst B, Ghia P, Niemann CU, Kater AP, Gregor M, Hallek M, Jerkeman M, Buske C. ESMO Guidelines Committee. ESMO clinical practice guideline interim update on new targeted therapies in the first line and at relapse of chronic lymphocytic leukaemia. Annals of Oncology. 2024;**35**(9):762–768

[35] Ciftciler R, Akın MG, Erat Z, Eşkazan AE. A systematic review on second Treatment-Free Remission (TFR) attempt in chronic myeloid leukemia (CML): Can it be applied in clinical practice? Clinical Lymphoma, Myeloma and Leukemia. 2023;**23**(1):8–14

[36] Özdemir Z N, Kılıçaslan NA, Yılmaz M, Eşkazan AE.Guidelines for the treatment of chronic myeloid leukemia from the NCCN and ELN: Differences and similarities. International Journal of Hematology. 2023;**17**(1):3–15

[37] Goldberg S, Hamarman S.Patients with chronic myelogenous leukaemia may not want to discontinue tyrosine kinase inhibitor therapy. Blood. 2015;**126**(23):1584–1584

[38] Richter J, Soderlund S, Lubking A, Dreimane A, Lotfi K, Markevarn B, et al Musculoskeletal pain in patients with chronic myeloid leukemia after discontinuation of imatinib: A tyrosine kinase inhibitor withdrawal syndrome? Journal of Clinical Oncology. 2014;**32**:2821–2823

[39] Mahon FX, Richter J, Guilhot J, Muller MC, Dietz C, Porkka K, Hjorth-Hansen H, Gruber F, Panagoitidis P, Ossenkoppele GJ, Mayer J.Interim analysis of a pan European stop tyrosine kinase inhibitor trial in chronic myeloid leukemia: The EURO-SKI study. Blood. 2014;**124**(21):151

[40] Rambhatla A, Strug MR, De Paredes JG, Cordoba Munoz MI, Thakur M.Fertility considerations in targeted biologic therapy with tyrosine kinase inhibitors: A review. Journal of Assisted Reproduction and Genetics. 2021;**38**(8):1897–1908

[41] Rosario R, Cui W, Anderson RA. Potential ovarian toxicity and infertility risk following targeted anti-cancer therapies. Reproduction and Fertility. 2022;**3**(3):R147–R162

[42] Robertson HF, Milojkovic D, Butt N, Byrne J, Claudiani S, Copland M, Gallipoli P, Innes AJ, Knight K, Mahdi AJ, Parker J. Expectations and outcomes of varying treatment strategies for CML presenting during pregnancy. British Journal of Haematology. 2024;**205**(3):947–955

[43] Assi R, Kantarjian H, Keating M, Pemmaraju N, Verstovsek S, Garcia-Manero G, Ravandi F, Borthakur G, Dahl J, Jabbour E, Cortes JE. Management of chronic myeloid leukemia during pregnancy among patients treated with a tyrosine kinase inhibitor: A single-center experience. Leukemia & Lymphoma. 2021;**62** (4):909917

[44] Tesch ME, Sorouri K, Zheng Y, Rosenberg SM, Ruddy KJ, Emmons KM, Dutton MC, Partridge AH. Contraception use and changes in young women with newly diagnosed breast cancer. Fertility and Sterility. 2025;**123** (3):488–498

[45] Elmakaty I, Saglio G, Al-Khabori M, Elsayed A, Elsayed B, Elmarasi M, Elsabagh AA, Alshurafa A, Ali E, Yassin M.The contemporary role of hematopoietic stem cell transplantation in the management of chronic myeloid leukemia: Is it the same in all settings? Cancers. 2024;**16**(4):754

[46] Niederwieser C, Morozova E, Zubarovskaya L, et al Risk factors for outcome after allogeneic stem cell transplantation in patients with advanced phase CML. Bone Marrow Transplantation. 2021;**56**:2834–2841

[47] Oyekunle A, Zander AR, Binder M, Ayuk F, Zabelina T, Christopeit M, et al Outcome of allogeneic SCT in patients with chronic myeloid leukemia in the era of tyrosine kinase inhibitor therapy. Annals of Hematology. 2013;**92**:487–496

Chapter 3

# Molecular Biological Insights into Large Granular Lymphocyte Leukemia

*Zou-Fang Huang and Jun Du*

## Abstract

Large granular lymphocytic leukemia (LGLL) represents a rare, indolent T-cell lymphoproliferative disorder. Clinically, it frequently manifests as cytopenia and organ infiltration. First-line immunosuppressive therapy induces clinical remission in approximately one-third to one-half of patients. Nevertheless, a significant proportion of patients experience a chronic disease course, necessitating long-term disease management. Precision medicine emerges as the pivotal future direction for this disease, with advances in molecular biology serving as the most potent driving force. In recent years, facilitated by the widespread adoption of next-generation sequencing technologies, the diagnostic and prognostic significance of gene mutations – such as those in STAT3 and STAT5B – has become increasingly elucidated within LGLL. These discoveries concurrently provide a rational foundation for exploring targeted therapeutic approaches, notably JAK inhibitors. However, the molecular landscape of LGLL remains substantially uncharted territory, warranting dedicated research efforts. This review synthesizes current progress in the molecular biology of LGLL, aiming to stimulate further investigation and offer insights for researchers in the field.

**Keywords:** large granular lymphocyte leukemia, molecular biology, indolent course, precision medicine, targeted therapy

## 1. Introduction

Large granular lymphocytic leukemia (LGLL) is a rare and indolent chronic hematologic malignancy characterized by the clonal proliferation of cytotoxic T cells or natural killer (NK) cells in the blood, bone marrow, and spleen. The clinical manifestations of LGLL are highly variable, ranging from asymptomatic cases to severe complications. Neutropenia is one of the most common presentations, occurring in 50–80% of patients. Affected individuals are prone to recurrent bacterial infections, such as skin infections, sinusitis, pneumonia, and oral ulcers. Severe neutropenia may lead to life-threatening sepsis.

Approximately 50% of patients develop anemia (a reduction in red blood cells), which may present with fatigue, weakness, dizziness, pallor, palpitations, and shortness of breath upon exertion. Some patients (about 20%) experience thrombocytopenia, manifesting as petechiae, bruising, epistaxis, gingival bleeding, or, in severe cases, visceral hemorrhage. A significant proportion of patients (around 30%) are asymptomatic at diagnosis, and their leukemic cell count may be very low. The disease typically follows an indolent course, and many cases are incidentally detected during routine blood tests performed for other reasons, prompted by persistent lymphocytosis or cytopenia.

LGLL is often associated with various autoimmune disorders, which may occasionally serve as the initial presenting manifestations; rheumatoid arthritis (RA) represents the most frequently observed comorbidity, with patients exhibiting symptoms such as symmetric joint pain, swelling, and morning stiffness closely resembling classic RA, while other autoimmune conditions such as systemic lupus erythematosus and autoimmune hemolytic anemia may also coexist. Additionally, a subset of patients experiences systemic "B symptoms" commonly associated with lymphoma, including unexplained fever (>38°C), drenching night sweats, and significant weight loss (exceeding 10% within 6 months). Splenomegaly is relatively common, occurring in 20–50% of cases and potentially leading to left upper quadrant abdominal fullness or discomfort, whereas hepatomegaly is less frequently encountered, and lymphadenopathy – generally mild and less prominent compared to other lymphomas – may also be present.

The first-line management of LGLL is primarily aimed at controlling symptoms, improving hematologic parameters, reducing clonal lymphocyte proliferation, and enhancing quality of life. For asymptomatic patients or those with only mild cytopenia and no signs of severe infections, a watch-and-wait approach with regular monitoring may be adopted instead of immediate active intervention. In cases requiring therapeutic intervention, immunosuppressive agents such as methotrexate, cyclophosphamide, and cyclosporine are commonly employed as first-line regimens. Only approximately half of patients derive clinical benefit from first-line immunosuppressive therapy. Most studies report a complete remission rate of about 20–30% and a partial remission rate of 20–40%. Notably, hematologic improvement is usually observed only after 2–4 months of treatment, and approximately 30–40% of patients experience relapse or drug resistance within 1–3 years. Notably, immunomodulatory therapy based on thalidomide has demonstrated promising efficacy; Chinese researchers have reported an overall response rate as high as 90% in preliminary clinical trials using the TPM regimen (thalidomide, prednisone, and methotrexate) for LGLL (NCT04453345) [1, 2], offering a novel therapeutic strategy for LGLL.

Despite its typically indolent course, a subset of patients with LGLL face refractory cytopenia and significant therapeutic challenges, underscoring the urgent need to elucidate its underlying molecular mechanisms. The T-LGLL clone comprises long-lived, activated, cytotoxic, and apoptosis-resistant T cells, which exhibit considerable heterogeneity across different patients [3]. The pathogenesis of LGLL is driven by persistent antigenic stimulation and constitutive activation of the JAK/STAT signaling pathway, coupled with a range of epigenetic alterations and resistance to apoptosis. LGLL originates from cytotoxic T cells or NK cells, which are typically involved in immune responses against viruses (such as EBV or CMV) or autoantigens. It is hypothesized that chronic antigen exposure serves as the initial driver of clonal selection, creating a selective pressure and microenvironment conducive to the acquisition of oncogenic mutations, such as those in STAT3. Elevated levels of inflammatory cytokines – including IL-15, IL-2, and IFN-γ – are frequently detected in patient sera. These cytokines not only activate the JAK/STAT pathway through their respective receptors but also foster a pro-inflammatory, pro-survival niche within the microenvironment that further supports the proliferation and survival of LGLL cells. These insights not only enhance the understanding of the disease mechanism but also open new avenues for targeted therapeutic interventions.

## 2. Narrative text

### 2.1 Driving mutations in the JAK/STAT signaling pathway

The JAK/STAT signaling pathway plays a critical role in regulating clonal development of T cells, and the presence of genetic mutations within this pathway serves as key evidence supporting clonal proliferation and confirming diagnosis. As early as 2001, researchers identified STAT3 mutations as central to LGLL pathogenesis, observing not only significantly elevated phosphorylation levels but also that inhibition using antisense oligonucleotides restored Fas/Fas-L-dependent apoptotic mechanisms [4]. Subsequent studies identified gain-of-function mutations in STAT3 in both T-cell and NK-cell variants of LGLL, elucidating a shared molecular mechanism between these two disease subtypes at the genetic level and providing compelling evidence for their classification under a single disease entity. According to large-scale clinical data, approximately 40–60% of T-LGLL and 30% of NK-LGLL cases harbor STAT3 mutations, a finding that establishes a critical rationale for molecularly targeted therapies [5].

Research has confirmed that STAT3 mutations represent the most prevalent driver alterations in T-LGLL and are also present in a subset of NK-LGLL patients. These mutations are typically missense variants located within the region encoding the Src homology 2 (SH2) domain, with the D661Y and Y640F mutations in the SH2 domain accounting for approximately 80% of these genetic changes [6]. The associated mutations lead to constitutive dimerization and phosphorylation of STAT3, resulting in upregulated transcription of anti-apoptotic genes (such as BCLXL and FLIP), cell-cycle-related genes (including CDKN1D and CMYC), as well as pro-inflammatory cytokine-encoding genes (e.g., IL-6, IL-12, IL-17, IL-21, IL-10, and IFN-γ) [7]. Notably, STAT3 mutations also exhibit significant heterogeneity, suggesting the potential presence of subclonal evolution within LGLL. From a clinical perspective, these gain-of-function mutations enhance T-cell cytotoxicity, which manifests as an increase in large granular lymphocytes in peripheral blood and subsequently leads to clinical features such as cytopenia.

In murine models, gain-of-function mutations in STAT3 induce the expansion of NKG2D$^+$CD8$^+$CD62L$^-$CD44$^+$ T cells, which subsequently upregulate cell cycle progression and expression of cytotoxic effector genes – such as GZMA and GZMB – via the NKG2D/IL-2–IL-15 signaling axis [8]. Furthermore, the clonal expansion of large granular lymphocytes may play a pivotal role in the pathogenesis and progression of autoimmune diseases, with LGL clones directly contributing to the proliferation of CD8$^+$ T lymphocytes [9]. Beyond mutational activation, the JAK/STAT pathway can also be dysregulated through non-mutational mechanisms, such as cytokine-mediated stimulation and epigenetic silencing of negative regulators – including microRNA-mediated modifications, with miR-181a and miR-146b implicated as potential contributors [10, 11].

Certainly, in addition to STAT3 mutations, STAT5B also represents a frequently mutated gene in this context, and both STAT3 and STAT5B mutations are significantly associated with clinical manifestations such as neutropenia and autoimmune features, including RA [12]. Building upon this, STAT5B mutations are observed in approximately 6% of γδ-T-LGLL cases, while their frequency rises strikingly to as high as 45% in the rarer indolent CD4-positive αβ-T-LGLL subtype [13]. Some researchers suggest that STAT5B gene mutations may be associated with a more aggressive clinical phenotype.

### 2.2 How do epigenetic alterations influence T-cell function?

Understanding the impact of epigenetic alterations on the clonal proliferation of T cells constitutes a critical foundation for advancing molecularly targeted therapies in LGLL. In the development of NK-LGLL, DNA methylation appears to be a key event, a view strongly supported by the high-frequency mutation of the TET2 gene – observed in approximately 28% to 34% of cases [14, 15]. It is important to emphasize, however, that TET2 mutations are not specific to LGLL and may also occur in age-related clonal hematopoiesis or clonal hematopoiesis of indeterminate potential. In the context of NK-LGLL, TET2 mutations drive an aberrant methylation pattern distinct from that of normal NK cells, characterized notably by hypermethylation of PTPRD – a key negative regulator of STAT3 – as well as SOCS3, a suppressor of JAK signaling; these epigenetic alterations collectively facilitate constitutive activation of the JAK/STAT pathway [16].

TET2 mutations can occur at an early stage and coexist simultaneously in both NK cells and myeloid cells. TET2 may promote clonal bias selection in NK cells, with the evolving clones subsequently acquiring STAT3 mutations, thereby exhibiting a cytotoxic NK-cell phenotype and ultimately leading to the development of clinically significant NK-LGLL. Supporting evidence includes the observation that approximately one-third of TET2-mutated cases also harbor concurrent STAT3 or CCL2 mutations. TET2 mutations may facilitate STAT3 activation through the epigenetic silencing of negative regulators of the JAK/STAT pathway [17]. Although TET2 mutations are also observed in T-LGLL, they appear to play a more pivotal role in the pathogenesis of NK-LGLL. This is evidenced by a more pronounced thrombocytopenia and a stronger association with malignant comorbidities.

Furthermore, in T-LGLL, mutations in the histone mono-methyltransferase KMT2D are observed in up to 20% of cases. While the precise role of KMT2D in the pathogenesis of LGLL remains elusive, chromatin accessibility analysis holds value in the differential diagnosis of mature T-cell malignancies [18].

Of particular note is that epigenetic modifications are increasingly emerging as a frontier in elucidating the pathogenesis of LGLL, where the application of single-cell multi-omics sequencing holds significant promise for unraveling the underlying molecular mechanisms.

### 2.3 CCL22 mutations are frequently identified in patients with NK-LGLL

Of particular significance is the observation that genetic alterations within the JAK/STAT signaling pathway extend beyond the canonical STAT3 and STAT5B mutations, with infrequent reports involving JAK1, JAK3, IL6R, PTPRT, and GNAS. Furthermore, mutations in genes such as NRAS, KRAS, PI3KCD, and TNFAIP3 also contribute to the genomic landscape of LGLL, though the pathogenic implications of many of these variants remain to be fully elucidated.

It has been reported that approximately 27% of NK-LGLL patients harbor mutations in the CCL22 coding gene, with these genetic alterations being correlated with an immunophenotype characterized by $CD16^{+}CD56^{bright}$ expression [19, 20]. These mutations are highly concentrated at evolutionarily conserved residue sites and exhibit mutual exclusivity with STAT3 mutations. CCL22 mutations represent gain-of-function alterations that result in defective CCR4 internalization in target cells, thereby enhancing cellular chemotaxis and disrupting normal interactions with the hematopoietic microenvironment. In vitro experiments demonstrate that myeloid and dendritic cells harboring CCL22 mutations produce elevated levels of IL-15, which drives clonal expansion of NK cells. Additionally, the cytokine CCL5, secreted by LGL clonal cells, induces monocytes to release high levels of IL-6, further promoting cellular proliferation [21]. However, there are currently no available drugs targeting CCL22, and research progress in this area remains limited.

### 2.4 Clonal hematopoiesis represents a pathogenic mechanism of critical importance that demands rigorous attention

A study by Shi M et al. revealed that T-cell clonopathy of undetermined significance (T-CUS) – defined as the detection of T-cell clonal expansion via high-sensitivity techniques in patients not meeting diagnostic criteria for lymphoma or leukemia – is a frequently encountered phenomenon in clinical practice, with a detection rate even higher than that of confirmed T-LGLL cases [22]. Patients with T-CUS and those diagnosed with T-LGLL exhibit highly overlapping features across multiple dimensions, including age, neutropenia, concomitant autoimmune disorders such as RA, and immunophenotypic profiles of clonal T cells – particularly the $CD8^{+}/CD57^{+}$ phenotype. Notably, driver gene mutations closely associated with T-LGLL, such as STAT3 mutations, have also been detected in a subset of T-CUS patients, challenging the conventional view that these genetic alterations are definitive markers of malignancy. These findings collectively indicate that the mere detection of T-cell clonality – or even the presence of a STAT3 mutation – can no longer be considered sufficient as absolute diagnostic criteria for T-LGLL. Rather, T-CUS and T-LGLL may represent different evolutionary stages within a single disease spectrum, rather than two distinct pathological entities.

The prevalence of clonal hematopoiesis (CH) is significantly higher in patients with LGLL compared to age-matched general populations, suggesting that the chronic immune stimulation, inflammatory milieu, or intrinsic biology of LGLL may provide a favorable niche for clonal expansion. A retrospective molecular analysis of 349 LGLL/T-CUS patients by Kawashima N et al. revealed CH in 19% of cases, with TET2 and DNMT3A mutations detected in 23% and 14% of patients, respectively. Multivariate analysis identified advanced age, splenomegaly, cytopenia, and STAT3/STAT5B mutations as factors positively associated with CH. Importantly, LGLL patients with CH exhibited a significantly elevated risk of developing myeloid neoplasms (10% vs. 2% at 5 years; $p = 0.02$), establishing CH as an independent adverse prognostic factor for both survival quality and secondary malignant transformation. CH may thus represent a "premalignant state" that heightens the risk of secondary oncogenesis.

Rather than a mere epiphenomenon, CH plays a pivotal role in LGLL pathogenesis, serving as both a critical prognostic biomarker and a potential therapeutic target. Routine screening for CH-associated gene mutations in LGLL patients could help identify high-risk subgroups prone to poor outcomes and secondary cancers, enabling closer monitoring and more aggressive clinical management.

### 2.5 Genetic mutations hold some, albeit limited, prognostic value in the context of disease outcomes

STAT3 mutations are strongly associated with the classic clinical features of LGLL, particularly neutropenia (which is both highly prevalent and severe), RA, and pure red cell aplasia (PRCA). Patients harboring STAT3 mutations demonstrate improved response rates to immunosuppressive therapies such as methotrexate, cyclophosphamide, and cyclosporine, allowing for more targeted therapeutic decision-making. Although STAT3 is recognized as a driver mutation, patients with these mutations exhibit relatively favorable overall survival (OS) compared to those with other molecular alterations, with a median survival often exceeding 10 years. Mortality risk is primarily attributed to severe infections secondary to neutropenia rather than direct transformation or progression of the disease itself.

STAT5B mutations, which are relatively uncommon (occurring in approximately 2–10% of cases) and most frequently represent gain-of-function alterations such as the N642H variant, constitute a well-established negative prognostic factor. These mutations are more prevalent in the $CD4^+$ T-LGLL subtype – as opposed to the more common $CD8^+$ phenotype – and are associated with a more aggressive clinical course, younger age of onset, splenomegaly, and overlapping features with other T-cell malignancies such as T-PLL. Patients with STAT5B mutations respond poorly to conventional first-line immunosuppressive therapies, often exhibiting limited clinical efficacy. Multiple studies have confirmed STAT5B mutations as an independent adverse prognostic marker, correlating with significantly shortened overall survival (OS). Affected individuals generally experience shorter survival times and a more aggressive disease phenotype.

Mutations in epigenetic regulators are present in over 40% of LGLL patients, often emerging prior to STAT3 mutations and regarded as "founding mutations" that shape disease progression and prognosis. Commonly affected genes include TET2, DNMT3A, and ASXL1 frequently associated with clonal hematopoiesis (CHIP-related mutations). The presence of these alterations is generally correlated with a more complex disease phenotype and diminished treatment response. In particular, patients harboring concurrent STAT3 and TET2 or DNMT3A mutations may require dual therapeutic targeting of both clonal hematopoiesis and LGLL, and typically exhibit a less favorable prognosis compared to those with STAT3 mutation alone.

Additionally, SF3B1 mutations are more frequently observed in LGLL patients with concomitant PRCA. While their independent prognostic significance remains under investigation, these mutations are generally associated with specific clinical subtypes.

Currently, STAT5B mutations represent a well-established negative prognostic marker in LGLL. In contrast, although STAT3 mutations are driver alterations, they are associated with a relatively "indolent" disease course and greater responsiveness to therapy. Co-occurring epigenetic mutations, such as those in TET2, further increase disease complexity and are indicative of a potentially poorer prognosis. Therefore, comprehensive genetic profiling – including STAT3, STAT5B, and a broader panel of accompanying mutations – has become an essential component of modern precision management for newly diagnosed LGLL patients. This approach not only facilitates accurate prognostic stratification but also provides critical guidance for treatment selection, suggesting, for example, that patients with STAT5B mutations may require more aggressive or innovative therapeutic strategies.

Emerging research has demonstrated that T-LGLL patients harboring STAT3 mutations exhibit significantly elevated surface CD38 expression on leukemic cells. Molecular studies have confirmed that activated STAT3 protein directly binds to the promoter region of the CD38 gene. The observed positive correlation between CD38 expression levels and STAT3 phosphorylation – a marker of activation – further supports a causal relationship between these two molecules. Given that STAT3 mutations directly drive CD38 overexpression, CD38 represents a highly promising therapeutic target in STAT3-mutated T-LGLL, as demonstrated by its direct transcriptional upregulation by STAT3. Theoretically, existing anti-CD38 monoclonal antibodies, such as daratumumab, could be leveraged to specifically recognize and eliminate these CD38-high leukemic cells [23]. Daratumumab binds to CD38 and mediates antibody-dependent cytotoxicity, complement activation, and phagocytosis, leading to selective depletion of $CD38^{+}$ leukemic clones. This approach represents a novel precision immunotherapy targeting the STAT3–CD38 axis in LGLL.

It is important to note that STAT3 and STAT5B mutations are hallmark driver alterations in LGLL. However, these mutations are occasionally also detected in the sequencing results of patients with myeloproliferative neoplasms (MPNs), such as MDS or MPN. This poses diagnostic challenges, as it remains clinically ambiguous whether such mutations originate from an underlying LGL clone or from the MPN itself. LGLL patients with STAT3 or STAT5B mutations typically exhibit a relatively straightforward mutational profile, often characterized by the presence of STAT3 or STAT5B alone or accompanied by a limited number of age-related clonal hematopoiesis (CHIP)-associated mutations, such as TET2 or DNMT3A. In contrast, MPN patients with coincident STAT3 or STAT5B mutations generally display a notably more complex molecular landscape, enriched with multiple driver mutations specific to myeloid malignancies – including ASXL1, SRSF2, U2AF1, JAK2, CALR, and MPL, among others [24]. Therefore, STAT3 and STAT5B mutations should not be interpreted in isolation. When these mutations are detected in a patient's bone marrow or peripheral blood samples, they must be evaluated within the broader mutational context. It is essential to recognize that LGLL is fundamentally characterized by an indolent clonal expansion of T or NK cells. A simple mutational profile supports the diagnosis of LGLL, whereas a complex genetic background – especially one enriched with characteristic mutations of myeloid neoplasms – favors a diagnosis of a myeloproliferative disorder.

### 2.6 Persistent activation of the JAK/STAT signaling pathway and its role in autoimmune pathogenesis

LGLL is fundamentally a clonal disorder, yet it is also intimately associated with autoimmune manifestations. These two aspects are intricately intertwined, collectively defining the disease phenotype. This autoimmune component is primarily driven by the constitutive activation of the STAT3 signaling pathway. STAT3 mutations are not only frequent driver events but also cause dysregulation of cytokine signaling – including IL-6, IL-15, and IL-21 – fostering a chronic inflammatory milieu. This environment supports the survival and expansion of

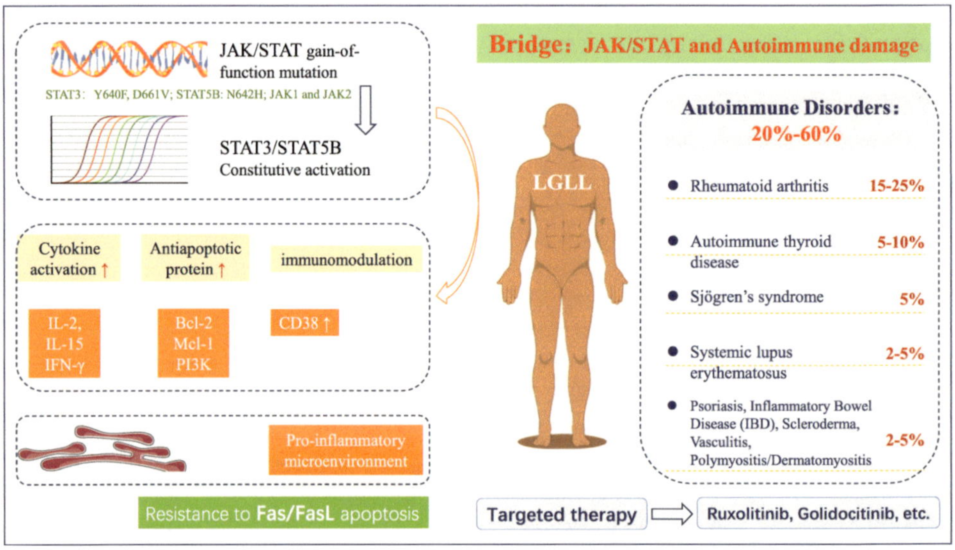


**Figure 1.**
*The JAK/STAT signaling pathway mediates autoimmune pathological injury in LGLL patients. Persistent antigenic stimulation and elevated cytokines (e.g., IL-6, IL-15, IL-21) activate the JAK/STAT pathway in cytotoxic T or NK cells. Gain-of-function mutations in STAT3 and STAT5B promote constitutive phosphorylation, dimerization, and nuclear translocation of STAT proteins, leading to transcriptional upregulation of anti-apoptotic (BCL-XL, MCL-1), pro-inflammatory (IL-6, IFN-γ, IL-21), and cell-cycle-related genes (MYC, CDKN1D). These events confer resistance to apoptosis, clonal expansion of cytotoxic lymphocytes, and overproduction of inflammatory cytokines that disrupt immune tolerance, resulting in autoimmune cytopenia and tissue injury. Therapeutically, JAK inhibitors can interrupt this pathogenic loop and restore immune homeostasis.*

leukemic cells while simultaneously disrupting immune tolerance, thereby promoting autoimmune attack [25].

Approximately one-third of patients with LGLL present with concomitant autoimmune diseases, most commonly RA. Correspondingly, first-line treatment for LGLL consists of oral immunosuppressive agents, reflecting a direct therapeutic targeting of its autoimmune nature. Targeted agents directed against key pathogenic mechanisms – particularly the JAK/STAT signaling pathway, such as JAK inhibitors – are emerging as promising therapeutic options, especially in relapsed or refractory cases. In a recent report by Hao H et al., a case of successful treatment of NK-LGLL with golidocitinib was described. The patient was a 53-year-old male diagnosed with NK-LGLL and harboring a STAT3 mutation. He had exhibited inadequate responses to multiple prior therapies, including methotrexate, cyclosporine, cyclophosphamide, thalidomide, and glucocorticoids. However, significant clinical improvement was achieved following treatment with the JAK1 inhibitor golidocitinib [26]. Not only was the patient's NK-LGLL effectively controlled, but a marked improvement was also observed in the concurrent hemolytic anemia. Therapy targeting the JAK/STAT signaling pathway thereby represents a novel and effective potential targeted strategy for managing this refractory condition, as illustrated in **Figure 1**.

## 3. Conclusion(s)

In summary, research on the molecular biology of LGLL has progressed from a purely descriptive discipline into an era of precision medicine grounded in signaling pathways and genetic mutations. The biological investigation of LGLL has transformed its diagnosis from a morphology-based nosology to a functional disorder driven by specific dysregulated signaling pathways. These molecular insights are not only of theoretical importance but are also poised to continually revolutionize precision diagnosis, risk stratification, and targeted therapy for LGLL. A deeper understanding of the JAK/STAT pathway mechanism represents a cornerstone in this field, offering new hope for disease control in affected patients.

LGLL is not a homogeneous disease; rather, diverse driver mutations define distinct subtypes with varying biological behaviors and clinical trajectories. Future research will remain focused on elucidating the disease origin, tracing clonal evolutionary history, and developing strategies to overcome resistance to targeted therapies. Patient mutation-informed animal and organoid models hold significant value for preclinical validation and novel drug exploration. Furthermore, given the immune characteristics of LGLL, whether immunotherapies such as CAR-T and bispecific antibodies hold potential for relapsed/refractory patients remains an open question worthy of further investigation.

## Acknowledgments

This work was funded by the Medical-Industrial Crossover Research Fund of Shanghai Jiao Tong University (China) and the "Jiao Tong University Star" Program (YG2024QNA13) (2024–2026).

## Conflict of interest

The authors declare no conflict of interest.

## Author details

Zou-Fang Huang[1] and Jun Du[2*]

1 Department of Hematology, Ganzhou Key Laboratory of Hematology, The First Affiliated Hospital of Gannan Medical University, Ganzhou, Jiangxi, China

2 Department of Hematology, Renji Hospital, School of Medicine, Shanghai Jiao Tong University, Shanghai, China

*Address all correspondence to: dujun-pathfinder@outlook.com

## References

[1] Yi S, Du J, Yu Y, Jiao Y, Wang Y, Wang H, Wang T, Lv R, Liu W, Xiong W, Liu H, Huang W, Zou D, An G, Zhao Y, Wang J, Qiu L. Thalidomide plus prednisone and methotrexate for symptomatic large granular lymphocyte leukemia: A prospective, single-center, pilot study. Blood. 2020;**136**:23–24

[2] Yu Y, Li Y, Cui R, Yan Y, Li F, Chen Y, Wang T, Hu X, Feng Y, Yu T, Huang Y, Sun J, Lyu R, Xiong W, Wang Q, Liu W, An G, Sui W, Xu Y, Huang W, Zou D, Wang H, Xiao Z, Wang J, Qiu L, Yi S. Thalidomide-based regimen shows promising efficacy in large granular lymphocytic leukemia: A multicenter phase II study. Signal Transduction and Targeted Therapy. 2025;**10**(1):85

[3] Gao S, Wu Z, Arnold B, Diamond C, Batchu S, Giudice V, Alemu L, Raffo DQ, Feng X, Kajigaya S, Barrett J, Ito S, Young NS. Single-cell RNA sequencing coupled to TCR profiling of large granular lymphocyte leukemia T cells. Nature Communications. 2022;**13**(1):1982

[4] Epling-Burnette PK, Liu JH, Catlett-Falcone R, Turkson J, Oshiro M, Kothapalli R, Li Y, Wang J-M, Yang-Yen H-F, Karras J, Jove R, Loughran Jr. TP. Inhibition of STAT3 signaling leads to apoptosis of leukemic large granular lymphocytes and decreased Mcl-1 expression. Journal of Clinical Investigation. 2001;**107**(3):351–362

[5] Lamy T, Pastoret C, Houot R, Ysebaert L, Hunault M, Damaj G, Banos A, Tournilhac O, Choufi B, Marolleau J-P, Dupuis J, Delmer A, Lepretre S, Gyan E, Feugier P, Rigaudeau S, Lazareth A, Malfuson J, Fest T, Bellissant E. Prospective, multicentric phase ii randomized trial comparing the efficacy of methotrexate or cyclophosphamide in large granular lymphocytic leukemia: A French National Study. Report on the interim analysis. Blood. 2019;**134**:1545–1545

[6] Jerez A, Clemente MJ, Makishima H, Koskela H, Leblanc F, Peng NK, Olson T, Przychodzen B, Afable M, Gomez-Segui I, Guinta K, Durkin L, Hsi ED, Mcgraw K, Zhang D, Wlodarski MW, Porkka K, Sekeres MA, List A, Mustjoki S, Loughran TP, Maciejewski JP. STAT3 mutations unify the pathogenesis of chronic lymphoproliferative disorders of NK cells and T-cell large granular lymphocyte leukemia. Blood. 2012;**120**(15):3048–3057

[7] Rajala HL, Olson T, Clemente MJ, Lagström S, Ellonen P, Lundan T, Hamm DE, Zaman SA, Lopez Marti JM, Andersson EI, Jerez A, Porkka K, Maciejewski JP, Loughran TP, Mustjoki S. The analysis of clonal diversity and therapy responses using STAT3 mutations as a molecular marker in large granular lymphocytic leukemia. Haematologica. 2015;**100**(1):91–99

[8] Masle-Farquhar E, Jackson KJL, Peters TJ, Al-Eryani G, Singh M, Payne KJ, Rao G, Avery DT, Apps G, Kingham J, Jara CJ, Skvortsova K, Swarbrick A, Ma CS, Suan D, Uzel G, Chua I, Leiding JW, Heiskanen K, Preece K, Kainulainen L, O'sullivan M, Cooper MA, Seppänen MRJ, Mustjoki S, Brothers S, Vogel TP, Brink R, Tangye SG, Reed JH, Goodnow CC. STAT3 gain-of-function mutations connect leukemia with autoimmune

disease by pathological NKG2D(hi) CD8 (+) T cell dysregulation and accumulation. Immunity. 2022;**55** (12):2386–2404.e8

[9] Mackie J, Ma CS, Tangye SG, Guerin A. The ups and downs of STAT3 function: Too much, too little and human immune dysregulation. Clinical and Experimental Immunology. 2023;**212**(2):107–116

[10] Assmann J, G LL, J SC, E VDBS, Schilperoord-Vermeulen J, Sandberg Y, Bellido M, J ES, J FD, P Jr LT. Langerak A W. miR-181a is a novel player in the STAT3-mediated survival network of TCRαβ+ CD8+ T large granular lymphocyte leukemia. Leukemia. 2022;**36**(4):983–993

[11] Mariotti B, Calabretto G, Rossato M, Teramo A, Castellucci M, Barilà G, Leoncin M, Vicenzetto C, Facco M, Semenzato G, Bazzoni F, Zambello R. Identification of a miR-146b-Fas ligand axis in the development of neutropenia in T large granular lymphocyte leukemia. Haematologica. 2020;**105**(5):1351–1360

[12] Fei F, Stehr H, Zehnder JL. Genomic landscape of T-large granular lymphocyte leukemia and chronic lymphoproliferative disorder of NK cells: A single institution experience. Leukemia & Lymphoma. 2023;**64** (9):1536–1544

[13] Muñoz-García N, Jara-Acevedo M, Caldas C, Bárcena P, López A, Puig N, Alcoceba M, Fernández P, Villamor N, Flores-Montero JA, Gómez K, Lemes MA, Hernández JC, Álvarez-Twose I, Guerra JL, González M, Orfao A, Almeida J. STAT3 and STAT5B mutations in T/NK-cell chronic lymphoproliferative disorders of large granular lymphocytes (LGL): Association with disease features. Cancers (Basel). 2020;**12**(12):3508

[14] Pastoret C, Desmots F, Drillet G, Le Gallou S, Boulland M-L, Thannberger A, Doncker A-V, Salaun V, Damaj GL, Veyrat-Masson R, Tournilhac O, Moignet A, Pangault C, Roussel M, Fest T, Lamy T. Linking the KIR phenotype with STAT3 and TET2 mutations to identify chronic lymphoproliferative disorders of NK cells. Blood. 2021;**137**(23):3237–3250

[15] Olson TL, Cheon H, Xing JC, Olson KC, Paila U, Hamele CE, Neelamraju Y, Shemo BC, Schmachtenberg M, Sundararaman SK, Toro MF, Keller CA, Farber EA, Onengut-Gumuscu S, Garrett-Bakelman FE, Hardison RC, Feith DJ, Ratan A, Loughran TP. Frequent somatic TET2 mutations in chronic NK-LGL leukemia with distinct patterns of cytopenias. Blood. 2021;**138**(8): 662–673

[16] Chan HW, Kurago ZB, Stewart CA, Wilson MJ, Martin MP, Mace BE, Carrington M, Trowsdale J, Lutz CT. DNA methylation maintains allele-specific KIR gene expression in human natural killer cells. Journal of Experimental Medicine. 2003;**197** (2):245–255

[17] Cheon H, Xing JC, Moosic KB, Ung J, Chan VW, Chung DS, Toro MF, Elghawy O, Wang JS, Hamele CE, Hardison RC, Olson TL, Tan S-F, Feith DJ, Ratan A, Loughran TP. Genomic landscape of TCRαβ and TCRγδ T-large granular lymphocyte leukemia. Blood. 2022;**139**(20): 3058–3072

[18] Julia E, Mareschal S, Chebel A, Golfier C, Müller T, Lours C, Hadj-Hamou S, Bissay N, Tschanz M,

Ceribelli M, Chartoire D, Vernay A, Sylvain C, Sibon D, Marçais A, Laurent C, Martin L, Asnafi V, Payen L, Bachy E. Chromatin accessibility profiling to increase diagnostic accuracy and refine cell-of-origin classification of mature T-cell lymphomas. Blood. 2021;**138**:809–809

[19] Baer C, Kimura S, Rana MS, Kleist AB, Flerlage T, Feith DJ, Chockley P, Walter W, Meggendorfer M, Olson TL, Cheon H, Olson KC, Ratan A, Mueller ML, Foran JM, Janke LJ, Qu C, Porter SN, S M P-M, Kalathur RC, Haferlach C, Kern W, Paietta E, Thomas PG, Babu MM, Loughran Jr. TP, Iacobucci I, Haferlach T, Mullighan CG. CCL22 mutations drive natural killer cell lymphoproliferative disease by deregulating microenvironmental crosstalk. Nature Genetics. 2022;**54**(5):637–648

[20] Mizuno Y, Kawakami T, Higano D, Miyairi S, Asakura A, Kawakami F, Sato K, Matsuzawa S, Nishina S, Sakai H, Higuchi Y, Matsuda K, Nakazawa H, Ishida F. CCL22 mutations in large granular lymphocytic leukemia. Haematologica. 2024;**109**(9):3067–3070

[21] Vicenzetto C, Gasparini VR, Barila G, Teramo A, Calabretto G, Rampazzo E, Carraro S, Trimarco V, Trentin L, Facco M, Semenzato G, Zambello R. Pro-inflammatory cells sustain leukemic clonal expansion in T-cell large granular lymphocyte leukemia. Haematologica. 2024;**109**(1):163–174

[22] Shi M, Olteanu H, Jevremovic D, He R, Viswanatha D, Corley H, Horna P. T-cell clones of uncertain significance are highly prevalent and show close resemblance to T-cell large granular lymphocytic leukemia. Implications for laboratory diagnostics. Modern Pathology. 2020;**33**(10):2046–2057

[23] Calabretto G, Buson E, Hutchins Z, Isabelle C, Scozzafava S, Trimarco V, Mariotti B, Burzinski R, Boles A, Rampazzo E, Teramo A, Manni S, Facco M, Barilà G, Bazzoni F, Semenzato G, Trentin L, Brammer JE, Zambello R, Mishra A. Activating STAT3 mutations drive CD38 expression in T-large granular lymphocytic leukemia. Blood. 2024;**144**:4132

[24] Kavesh M, Mohebnasab M, Angel MR, Xie W, Raess PW, Cui W, Press RD, Yang G, Li P. Distinguishing STAT3/STAT5B -mutated large granular lymphocyte leukemia from myeloid neoplasms by genetic profiling. Blood Advances. 2023;**7**(1):40–45

[25] Marchand T, Pastoret C, Moignet A, Roussel M, Lamy T. Large granular lymphocyte leukemia: A clonal disorder with autoimmune manifestations. Hematology: American Society of Hematology Education Program. 2024;**2024**(1):143–149

[26] Hao H, Yuan C, Zhang C, Jian J. Golidocitinib was used for the first time to treat refractory NK-Large Granular lymphocytic leukemia with a STAT3 mutation, accompanied by hemolytic anemia: A case report. Frontiers in Immunology. 2025;**16**:1632803

[27] Zhang L, Qiu C, Li R, Shen Y, Tian L, Chang H, Liang Q, Pan H, Gao Z, Li W, Zhao J, Fang L, Yu X, Xu J, Kuang Z, Yuan W, Chu Y, Shi J. KLRG1 re-defines a leukemic clone of CD8 effector T cells sensitive to PI3K inhibitor in T cell large granular lymphocytic leukemia. Cell Reports Medicine. 2025;**6**(4):102036

Chapter 4

# Leukemia and the Eye: Ocular Manifestations, Diagnosis and Therapeutic Approaches

*Alan Chew-Bonilla, Emiliano Fulda Graue, Jorge Morales-Navarro, Maria Renee Jimenez-Sotomayor and Federico Graue Wiechers*

## Abstract

Leukemia comprises a heterogeneous group of hematologic malignancies characterized by uncontrolled proliferation of abnormal leukocytes, leading to bone marrow failure and systemic manifestations. Ocular involvement is common and may represent the first sign of disease, relapse, or systemic progression. The eye, considered an extension of the central nervous system, is susceptible to direct leukemic infiltration as well as secondary effects from hematologic abnormalities and treatment complications. Clinical manifestations range from anterior segment signs such as conjunctival infiltration, pseudohypopyon, and hyphema to posterior segment findings including retinal hemorrhages, cotton-wool spots, venous tortuosity, and serous retinal detachment due to choroidal infiltration. Orbital involvement, particularly in pediatric acute leukemias, can present with myeloid sarcoma, leading to unilateral or bilateral proptosis and diplopia. Optic nerve infiltration represents a neuro-oncologic emergency with potentially irreversible visual loss if untreated. Diagnosis requires a multidisciplinary approach involving complete ophthalmic examination, multimodal imaging, and occasionally tissue biopsy. Management is primarily systemic chemotherapy. Ocular involvement carries significant prognostic implications, correlating with higher relapse rates and reduced survival. Early recognition of ocular signs by ophthalmologists is critical for timely diagnosis, systemic evaluation, and initiation of appropriate therapy, which may preserve vision and improve overall outcomes.

**Keywords:** leukemia, ocular manifestations, choroidal infiltration, optic nerve involvement, orbital infiltration

## 1. Introduction

**Leukemia** represents a heterogeneous group of malignant hematologic neoplasms originating from the abnormal and dysfunctional proliferation of developing leukocytes or hematopoietic stem cells in the bone marrow. This uncontrolled expansion of immature cells disrupts normal hematopoiesis, compromising the production of healthy blood cells and resulting in a wide spectrum of clinical manifestations [1].

Ocular involvement is more common in acute leukemias than in chronic ones, and more frequently in the myeloid than the lymphoid variant. Reported prevalence ranges between 32% and 35% in clinical series, although histopathological studies suggest intraocular involvement in up to 90% of cases [2].

Leukemia classification is based on proliferation rate and cell type. Acute forms, defined by more than 20% blasts in bone marrow or blood, evolve rapidly and can be fatal within months if untreated. Chronic forms have less than 20% blasts, progress slowly, and feature partially mature but ineffective cells.

According to the cell lineage of origin, the disease may be myeloid or lymphoid. Combining both criteria yields the four classic subtypes:

- **Acute lymphoblastic leukemia (ALL):** blast transformation of lymphoid progenitors (B or T), representing up to 80% of cases in the pediatric population.

- **Acute myeloid leukemia (AML):** defined by more than 20% myeloid blasts, is the most common acute form in adults and typically has an aggressive course.

- **Chronic lymphocytic leukemia (CLL):** proliferation of monoclonal lymphocytes predominates between 60 and 70 years of age and usually follows an indolent course.

- **Chronic myeloid leukemia (CML):** associated with the reciprocal BCR-ABL1 translocation, which gives rise to the Philadelphia chromosome and leads to the expansion of dysfunctional granulocytes [1].

From an epidemiological standpoint, leukemia ranks tenth among the most common cancers in the United States of America, with approximately 61,000 new cases annually. Its etiology is multifactorial, including genetic predisposition (syndromes such as Down, Klinefelter, Bloom, Li-Fraumeni), germline mutations in genes such as RUNX1 or CEBPA, viral infections (Epstein–Barr, HTLV-1), as well as exposure to ionizing radiation, benzene, smoking, and prior chemotherapy.

Initial symptoms are often nonspecific: fever, fatigue, weight loss, bone pain, anemia and hemorrhagic syndromes, as well as signs of systemic infiltration such as hepatosplenomegaly or lymphadenopathy [1].

**Ocular manifestations of Leukemia**

Ophthalmological manifestations are highly relevant, as they may constitute the first evidence of the disease, a relapse, or systemic progression. The eye, considered an extension of the central nervous system, allows direct infiltration by leukemic cells and makes therapeutic control more challenging.

Two main pathophysiological mechanisms are distinguished:

- **Direct leukemic infiltration:** invasion of ocular and orbital tissues by blasts.

- **Secondary involvement:** resulting from hematologic alterations (anemia, thrombocytopenia, hyperviscosity) or from complications of chemotherapy and immunosuppression (opportunistic infections) [2].

**Diagnosis and treatment**

Diagnosis requires interdisciplinary collaboration. A complete blood count (CBC) with differential and the presence of blasts in peripheral blood raise suspicion, confirmed by a bone marrow aspirate and biopsy. A lumbar puncture assesses CNS involvement, which may be negative even with ocular infiltration.

The treatment of ocular manifestations is based on the systemic control of leukemia:

- **Systemic chemotherapy:** the therapeutic cornerstone, is used with regimens tailored to the leukemia subtype.
- **Immunotherapy:** particularly useful in cases of minimal residual disease or relapses.
- **Local radiotherapy:** reserved for refractory cases, though it carries the risk of ocular toxicity (retinopathy, cataracts).
- **Hematopoietic stem cell transplantation:** indicated in high-risk scenarios or relapses.
- **Adjunctive therapies:** (leukapheresis, hydroxyurea) in the context of hyper-leukocytosis [1].

## 2. Orbital involvement in leukemia

The orbit can be affected during the course of leukemia, although orbital leukemic infiltration is considered relatively uncommon. Its incidence in the pediatric population ranges from 2% to 13%, being more frequent in acute leukemias (ALL and AML) than in chronic forms.

In children, the orbit is one of the most common sites of presentation, and it is estimated that 2% to 6% of orbital tumors in childhood correspond to leukemia. Orbital involvement is also associated with a poorer prognosis and a higher risk of relapse.

**Clinical manifestations**

AML can initially present with orbital involvement, even before the underlying leukemia is diagnosed. The accumulation of leukemic cells in soft tissues – previously referred to as granulocytic sarcoma – is now termed **myeloid sarcoma** [3]. This entity occurs in 2.5–9.1% of patients with AML [4]. Unilateral proptosis is the predominant sign, sometimes accompanied by ptosis, eyelid edema, decreased visual acuity, and diplopia. Bilateral involvement, although less common, is considered a clinical marker of high-risk myeloid sarcoma. The typical location is superior or superotemporal [5], and there may be involvement of the lacrimal gland and extraocular muscles.

Other, less common presentations have been reported, such as acute dacryocystitis secondary to leukemic infiltration [6], or diffuse eyelid thickening with eyelid swelling [7].

**Diagnosis**

Diagnosis requires a multidisciplinary approach. A complete ophthalmic examination is the first step, complemented by imaging studies:

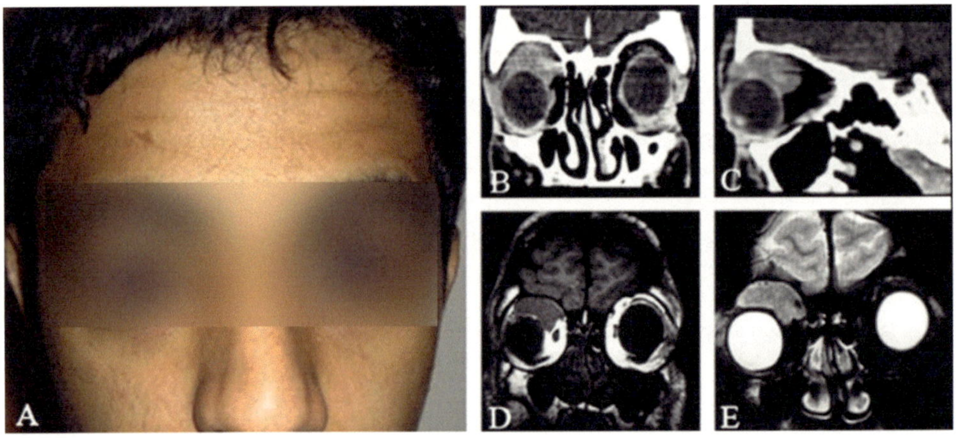


**Figure 1.**
*(a) External photograph of a 17-year-old male showing right upper eyelid swelling, downward displacement of his right eye globe, and proptosis; (b and c) computed tomography scan (coronal and sagittal views); and (d and e) magnetic resonance imaging (coronals T1WI and T2WI) demonstrate an evidence of a uniform, well-demarcated lesion occupying the superior orbit and compressing the globe downward and outward. Complete excision of the tumor and histopathologic diagnosis revealed evidence of acute myeloid leukemia (AML).*


**Magnetic resonance imaging (MRI) of the orbits and brain:** useful to rule out compressive lesions and to assess local extension. On T1-weighted images, orbital masses appear isointense relative to gray matter and muscle, while on T2-weighted images, the masses are isointense relative to white matter and muscle [5] (**Figure 1**).

**Computed tomography (CT):** orbital leukemic involvement appears as a well-defined, homogeneous mass, isodense or hyperdense compared to brain tissue, with mild homogeneous enhancement after contrast injection. It may arise in either an intraconal or extraconal location. The mass molds to the bone and orbital structures [4].

**Orbital biopsy:** indicated when clinical and imaging findings are inconclusive or when the orbital lesion is the only apparent manifestation of leukemia. Thanks to advances in imaging techniques and the understanding of hematologic neoplasms, we no longer have to rely as frequently on confirmatory biopsies to establish the diagnosis of leukemic tumors [5].

**Treatment**

Management focuses on systemic control of the underlying leukemia through chemotherapy. In selected cases – such as the development of compressive optic neuropathy despite systemic chemotherapy – local radiotherapy may be necessary [5].

## 3. Anterior segment involvement

Manifestations in the anterior segment are less frequent than those in the posterior segment but can become clinically significant and, in some cases, represent the initial presentation of leukemia.

**Conjunctiva**

Conjunctival infiltration is rarely encountered in acute leukemia. An autopsy study reported conjunctival involvement in 4% of leukemia patients [8]. It appears as a raised, fleshy, salmon-colored mass. Conjunctival myeloid sarcoma is rare but has been described in the literature. Bilateral subconjunctival hemorrhages have also been reported as an initial manifestation of AML. In CLL, venous "comma-shaped" irregularities can be seen, probably secondary to hyperviscosity.

**Cornea**

Because of its avascular nature, the cornea is rarely a site of direct leukemic infiltration. However, cases of sterile ring corneal ulcer with iritis and pannus as an initial presentation of AML have been reported [9]. Chemotherapy-related epithelial changes, such as corneal thinning, may also be observed [10].

**Anterior chamber**

Pseudohypopyon is a rare manifestation at AML onset but is more frequently observed in recurrent disease. In pediatric ALL, it may occur in up to 2.5% of relapses. Leukemic hypopyon is often associated with extramedullary infiltration, particularly of the CNS, although isolated ocular relapse has been reported. Another possible manifestation is increased intraocular pressure due to trabecular infiltration [11]. In pediatric patients, leukemia can also be a cause of spontaneous hyphema [8].

**Iris**

Iris infiltration often coexists with choroidal and ciliary body involvement and is not always clinically apparent. When it does manifest, it may cause changes in iris coloration [8].

**Diagnosis**

Diagnosis requires a comprehensive approach. Slit-lamp examination is essential for detecting conjunctival, corneal, or inflammatory lesions.

**Conjunctival biopsy:** although ocular manifestations of leukemia are rarely biopsied, conjunctival biopsy can be a useful diagnostic procedure to identify the etiology of lesions, particularly when clinical and imaging findings are inconclusive or when ocular manifestations represent the initial symptom [12]. Lesions can sometimes be the first sign of the primary disease or of relapse, even in the absence of documented systemic recurrence [11].

**Anterior chamber paracentesis with cytology and flow cytometry studies**: recommended when leukemic or tumoral infiltration is suspected, particularly if pseudohypopyon or visible cells are present [13].

**Treatment**

The cornerstone of management is systemic leukemia control with chemotherapy.

## 4. Retinal and choroidal involvement

The retina and choroid are the most commonly affected ocular tissues in leukemia [14]. Up to 90% of patients are estimated to present with fundus abnormalities at some point during their disease course. Posterior segment involvement is associated with a worse systemic prognosis and a higher risk of bone marrow or CNS relapse.

**Retina**

Retinal hemorrhages are the most frequent manifestation of leukemic retinopathy [2, 15]. They can appear in different forms: dot-and-blot, flame-shaped, preretinal,

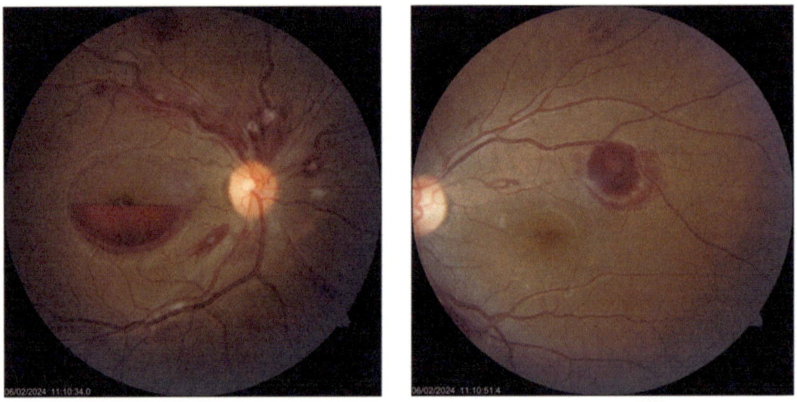

**Figure 2.**
*Fundus picture of the right eye showing Roth spots and subhyaloid hemorrhage at the macula, and fundus picture of the left eye showing Roth spots.* ***CC BY–NC–SA 4.0.***

subretinal, or subhyaloid hemorrhages. Roth spots – hemorrhages with a white center – are characteristic and result from capillary rupture with fibrin–platelet thrombus formation, sometimes with accumulation of leukemic cells. Macular involvement can cause significant visual impairment [2] (**Figure 2**). In AML, the presence of intraretinal hemorrhages correlates closely with thrombocytopenia.

Cotton-wool spots occur due to the occlusion of precapillary arterioles and consequent retinal nerve fiber layer ischemia or focal leukemic infiltrates. In acute leukemia, their presence is associated with a poor prognosis, increasing three-month mortality up to eightfold [16].

Leukemic infiltrates have diverse clinical presentations, including large whitish-gray nodules of various sizes in the retina, whitish-gray streaks along vessels from perivascular infiltrates, subretinal infiltrates, optic nerve infiltration, choroidal infiltrates leading to serous retinal detachment, retinal pigment epithelium detachments, and vitreous infiltrates. These are associated with elevated leukocytosis and local tissue damage [17].

Blood hyperviscosity can result in vascular tortuosity and central retinal vein or artery occlusions [15]. Vascular sheathing may also occur due to perivascular blast infiltration [17]. Peripheral microaneurysms – more common in chronic leukemias – have been reported [17]. Peripheral neovascularization resembling sickle-cell retinopathy can occur in CML, associated with chronic leukocytosis [17].

**Choroid**

The choroid is one of the most commonly infiltrated sites by leukemic cells, often subclinically. Postmortem histopathological studies report choroidal infiltration in up to 65% of patients and in 31% of eyes from patients who died of leukemia. This involvement is more common in relapse settings and is usually associated with systemic and CNS disease [18].

Serous retinal detachment is the most frequent clinical manifestation of choroidal infiltration. It is attributed to choroidal hypoperfusion and retinal pigment epithelium dysfunction, with disruption of the outer blood–retinal barrier. It has been documented as the initial presentation of AML in both adults and children [19].

**Diagnosis**

Diagnosis requires a complete ophthalmic examination with pupillary dilation.

- **Optical coherence tomography (OCT):** crucial for identifying subfoveal serous detachments and measuring choroidal thickness, which may be increased, suggesting infiltration. EDI-OCT (enhanced depth imaging OCT) allows precise evaluation of the choroid. OCT also documents intraretinal, sub-ILM hemorrhages, and macular structural changes.

- **Fluorescein angiography:** may demonstrate a multifocal leakage pattern within the macular area [19].

**Treatment**

The mainstay of therapy is systemic leukemia control, which resolves leukemic retinopathy in most cases. However, local or adjunctive interventions have been reported in cases of persistent vitreoretinal infiltration despite systemic therapy [15].

- **Intravitreal methotrexate:** evaluated in intraocular infiltration; while visual acuity did not change, anterior chamber inflammation decreased, optic disc edema resolved, and tumor cell infiltrates were absorbed. However, it has not been shown to resolve retinal hemorrhages [13].

- **Pars plana vitrectomy:** indicated for persistent vitreous hemorrhage, vitreomacular traction, or tractional retinal detachment [20].

**Prognostic implications**

Posterior segment involvement correlates with a worse systemic prognosis. In particular, the presence of leukemic retinopathy at diagnosis is associated with a five-year survival rate of 21.4%, compared with 45.7% in patients without ocular involvement. Cotton-wool spots, specifically, are strongly associated with increased mortality [21].

## 5. Neuro-ophthalmologic manifestations

Optic nerve infiltration by leukemia or lymphoma constitutes a neuro-oncologic emergency. Postmortem studies have demonstrated optic nerve involvement in up to 18% of acute leukemias and 16% of chronic leukemias, with higher prevalence in ALL and pediatric patients [8].

Leukemic optic neuropathy can result from direct leukemic cell infiltration of the optic nerve head or retrolaminar portion, CNS infiltration with raised intracranial pressure presenting as papilledema, or local extension of blasts causing retrolaminar invasion [22].

Although it is often accompanied by other neurologic or systemic findings, optic nerve infiltration can occasionally be the first sign of relapse [22].

In children, ALL is the most common cause of isolated infiltrative neuropathy (≈75% of cases), followed by B-cell non-Hodgkin lymphoma. In adults, it has been reported with ALL, AML, CLL, and CML [22].

**Clinical manifestations**

Presentation is variable, but the most common symptoms are rapidly progressive visual loss, retro-ocular pain or pain with eye movements, optic disc edema – typically accompanied by hemorrhages – diplopia, or cranial nerve palsies when there is involvement of oculomotor nerves [23]. Associated neurologic symptoms, such as nausea, vomiting, lethargy, or seizures, may occur in the context of CNS involvement (**Figures 3** and **4**).

**Diagnosis**

A thorough, multimodal diagnostic approach is required:

Complete ophthalmic examination with visual acuity assessment, pupillary examination (looking for a relative afferent pupillary defect), and fundus evaluation for disc edema, hemorrhages, or perivascular infiltrates.

**Brain and orbital MRI:** essential to exclude compressive lesions and assess dissemination. It may show optic nerve thickening and enhancement, with T2 hyperintensity or restricted diffusion; however, findings can be normal in some cases.

**CT scan:** may reveal optic nerve thickening and enhancement.

**Lumbar puncture with cerebrospinal fluid analysis:** may be required to detect CNS involvement, although CSF can be negative even in the presence of optic nerve infiltration [22].

**Treatment**

Management must be initiated urgently to preserve vision:

- **Systemic corticosteroids:** may facilitate rapid visual recovery, but early administration can mask clinical and pathological findings, making diagnosis more challenging. Intravenous methylprednisolone pulse therapy, followed by a tapering course of oral prednisone, has been used [22].

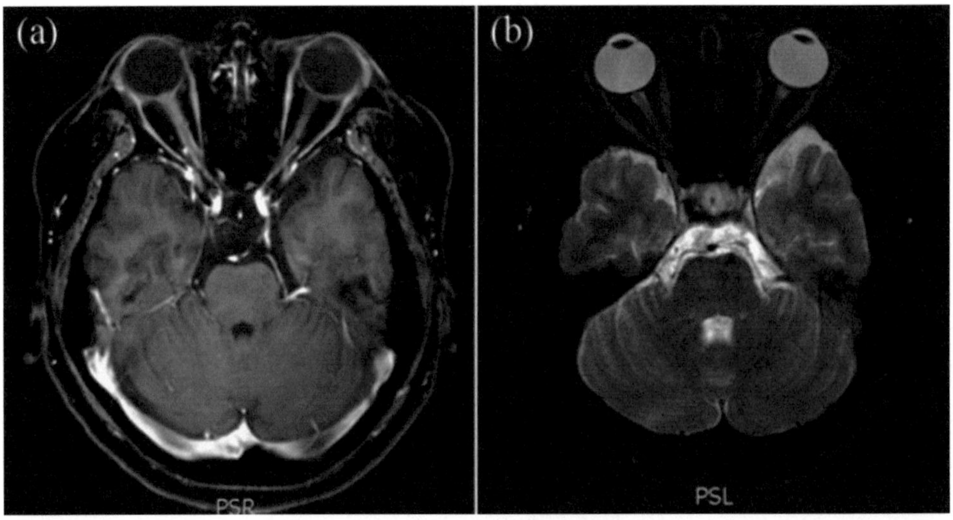


**Figure 3.**
*(a) MRI T1-weighted brain and orbits. Surrounding the right optic nerve, pronounced gadolinium uptake can be seen. (b) MRI orbit scan repeated after completion of therapy. The right optic nerve is no longer thickened.*

*DOI: http://dx.doi.org/10.5772/intechopen.1013644*

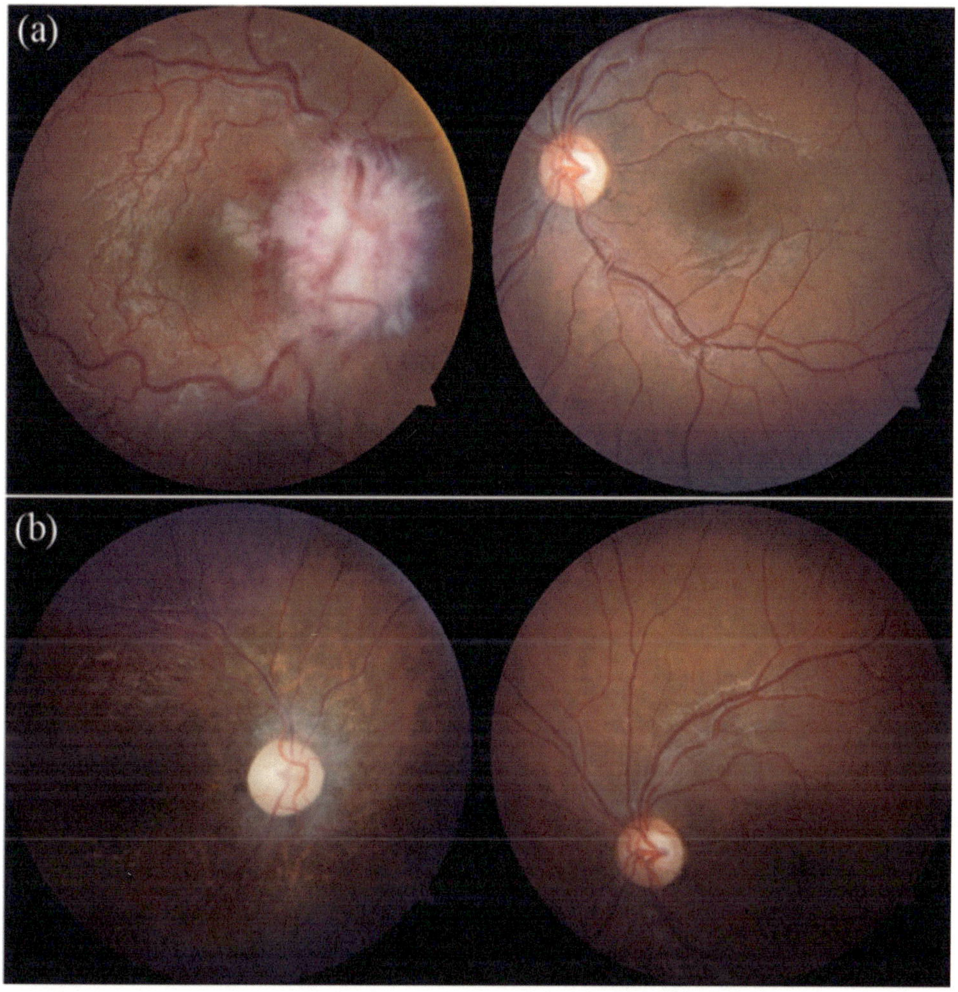


**Figure 4.**
*(a) Fundus photographs at initial presentation: right eye and left eye, respectively. The left eye was normal, while the right showed significant disc edema, tortuosity of the retinal vessels and hemorrhages. (b) Fundus photographs of the right and left eye, 3 months following bone marrow transplant. Resolution of disc edema can be noted.*

### Prognosis

Optic nerve infiltration in leukemia is a marker of poor prognosis, associated with higher rates of bone marrow relapse and CNS involvement. Visual loss may be severe and irreversible despite prompt treatment [11].

A 14-year-old male with T-cell ALL in remission presented with the sudden onset of right eye pain and visual acuity impairment.

Fundoscopic examination of the eye and MRI of the orbits were consistent with optic nerve infiltration. The patient was treated with salvage chemotherapy, orbital radiation, and eventual bone marrow transplantation, with notable improvement in vision and regression of retinal and optic nerve findings. **CC BY–NC 4.0.**

## 6. Conclusion(s)

Management of ocular leukemia relies primarily on systemic chemotherapy to control the underlying disease. Multidisciplinary collaboration between hematologists, oncologists, and ophthalmologists is essential for accurate diagnosis, timely treatment, and preservation of vision. Awareness of the diverse spectrum of ocular presentations and their prognostic implications can improve patient outcomes and support comprehensive care for individuals with leukemia.

## Conflict of Interest

The authors declare no conflict of interest.

## Author details

Alan Chew-Bonilla*, Emiliano Fulda Graue, Jorge Morales-Navarro, Maria Renee Jimenez-Sotomayor and Federico Graue Wiechers
Conde de Valenciana Institute of Ophthalmology, Mexico City, Mexico

*Address all correspondence to: alanchewbonilla@gmail.com

## References

[1] Chennamadhavuni A, Iyengar V, Mukkamalla SKR, et al. Leucemia. [Actualizado el 17 de enero de 2023]. StatPearls. Internet. Isla del Tesoro (FL): StatPearls Publishing; 2025. enero-. Disponible en https://www.ncbi.nlm.nih.gov/books/NBK560490/

[2] Yan B, Luo L, Shen J, Huang Y. Secondary ocular manifestations in acute leukemia: Clinical patterns and hematologic correlates. Journal of Multidisciplinary Healthcare. 2025;**18**:3289–3297. DOI: 10.2147/jmdh.s522369

[3] Shields JA, Stopyra GA, Marr BP, et al. Sarcoma mieloide orbitario bilateral como signo inicial de leucemia mieloide aguda: Informe de caso y revisión de la literatura. Archives of Ophthalmology. 2003;**121**(1):138. DOI: 10.1001/archopht.121.1.138

[4] Razem B, Raiteb M, El Mrini S, Slimani F. 2021. Orbital myeloid sarcoma misdiagnosed for subperiostal hematoma: A case report. Journal of Medical Case Reports. **15**(1):501. DOI: 10.1186/s13256-021-03025-8

[5] Bidar M, Wilson MW, Laquis SJ, Wilson TD, Fleming JC, Wesley RE, Ribeiro RC, Haik BG. 2007. Clinical and imaging characteristics of orbital leukemic tumors. Ophthalmic Plastic and Reconstructive Surgery. **23**(2): 87–93. DOI: 10.1097/iop.0b013e3180333a85

[6] Wirostko WJ, Garcia GH, Cory S, Harris GJ. 1999. Acute dacryocystitis as a presenting sign of pediatric leukemia. American Journal of Ophthalmology. **127**(6):734–736. DOI: 10.1016/s0002-9394(99)00023-9

[7] Mirshahi R, Ghassemi F, Koochakzadeh L, Faranoush M, Ghomi Z, Mehrvar A, Mousavi SA, Nodehi SRS. 2022. Ocular manifestations of newly diagnosed acute leukemia patients. Journal of Current Ophthalmology. **34**(1): 100–105. DOI: 10.4103/joco.joco_10_21

[8] Kincaid MC, Green WR. Ocular and orbital involvement in leukemia. Survey of Ophthalmology. 1983;**27**:211–232

[9] Wood WJ, Nicholson DH. 1973. Corneal ring ulcer as the presenting manifestation of acute monocytic leukemia. American Journal of Ophthalmology. **76**(1):69–72. DOI: 10.1016/0002-9394(73)90013-5

[10] Sharma T, Grewal J, Gupta S, Murray PI. 2004. Ophthalmic manifestations of acute leukaemias: The ophthalmologist's role. Eye. **18**(7): 663–672. DOI: 10.1038/sj.eye.6701308

[11] El Salloukh NA, Hage DG, Bashshur AZ, Kheir WJ. Early ophthalmological manifestations of acute myeloid leukemia: Current perspectives. <![CDATA[Clinical Ophthalmology]]>. 2022;**16**:2119–2127. DOI: 10.2147/OPTH.S342720

[12] Chakroborty K, Hasan MM, Hasanuzzaman M, Sultana Z, Khaleque SA. 2024. Ophthalmic manifestations of leukemia and their management. Mugda Medical College Journal. 7(1):36–41. DOI: 10.3329/mumcj.v7i1.73969

[13] Vishnevskia-Dai V, Sella King S, Lekach R, et al. Ocular manifestations of leukemia and results of treatment with

intravitreal methotrexate. Scientific Reports. 2020;**10**:1994

[14] De Queiroz Mendonca C, Freire MV, Viana SS, Tavares MKGS, Silva WMA, Cipolotti R. Ocular manifestations in acute lymphoblastic leukemia: A five-year cohort study of pediatric patients. Leukemia Research. 2018;**76**:24–28. DOI: 10.1016/j.leukres.2018.11.017

[15] Beketova T, Mordechaev E, Murillo B, Schlesinger MD. Leukemic retinopathy: A diagnostic clue for initial detection and prognosis of leukemia. Cureus. 2023. DOI: 10.7759/cureus.50587

[16] Abu El-asrar AM, Al-momen AK, Kangave D, Harakati MS. Prognostic importance of retinopathy in acute leukemia. Documenta Ophthalmologica. 1995;**91**:273–281. DOI: 10.1007/BF01204178

[17] Maniam A, Zuhaimy H, Vendargon FMM, Othman O. 2021. Isolated ocular manifestations in chronic myeloid leukaemia. Cureus. **13**(11):e19450. DOI: 10.7759/cureus.19450

[18] Yang L, Chen Y, Zhang Y, Shen T, Shen X. Changes in retinal circulation and choroidal thickness in patients with acute myeloid leukemia detected by optical coherence tomography angiography. Frontiers in Medicine (Lausanne). 2023;**10**. 1117204. DOI: 10.3389/fmed.2023.1117204

[19] Adaniya A, Luciano AD, Alvarado-Villacorta R, Saravia MJ, Morales-Cantón V, Bazterrechea P, Schlaen BA. 2022. Serous retinal detachment as a sign of leukemic choroidopathy: A systematic review. Survey of Ophthalmology. **67**(1):149–167. DOI: 10.1016/j.survophthal.2021.04.007

[20] Kudo T, Suzuki Y, Metoki T, Nakazawa M. 2015. A case of childhood vitrectomy performed for dense vitreous hemorrhage secondary to leukemia therapy and tumor lysis syndrome. Case Reports in Ophthalmology. **6**(1):34–38. DOI: 10.1159/000374088

[21] Ohkoshi K, Tsiaras WG. 1992. Prognostic importance of ophthalmic manifestations in childhood leukaemia. British Journal of Ophthalmology. **76**(11):651–655. DOI: 10.1136/bjo.76.11.651

[22] Myers KA, Nikolic A, Romanchuk K, Weis E, Brundler M, Lafay-Cousin L, Costello F. 2016. Optic neuropathy in the context of leukemia or lymphoma: Diagnostic approach to a neuro-oncologic emergency. Neuro-Oncology Practice. **4**(1):60–66. DOI: 10.1093/nop/npw006

[23] Gong J, Li J, Liang H. 2011. Extramedullary relapse presenting as trigeminal neuralgia and diplopia after allogeneic hematopoietic stem cell transplantation. Internal Medicine. **50**(10):1117–1119. DOI: 10.2169/internalmedicine.50.4909

Chapter 5

# New Approaches to the Treatment of Chronic Myeloid Leukemia

*Lyudmyla P. Shvachko, Svitlana Antonenko, Michael Zavelevich, Irene Gartovska, Mykhailo Dybkov, Dmytro Gur`yanov and Gennadii Telegeev*

## Abstract

While the specific inhibitors of BCR-ABL tyrosine kinase activity have gained well-deserved recognition in the frontline therapy of chronic myeloid leukemia (CML), acquired therapy resistance represents a serious problem, preventing long-term remission in CML patients. Moreover, in some patients, the resistance mechanisms are BCR-ABL-independent. Therefore, the search for alternative and complementary therapies is currently in the spotlight. The differentiation therapy may represent one of the possible approaches. Alpha-tocopherol may be one of the agents possessing differentiation potential in CML blast cells. We demonstrated that alpha-tocopherol and G-CSF upregulate the expression of several genes associated with the differentiation of K562 CML cells in vitro, in particular, the gene coding for the myeloid master regulator transcription factor C/EBPα. At the same time, a significant down-regulation of the expression of genes associated with the stemness phenotype, such as *SNAI1, ALPP*, and *POU5F1* was observed. Other possible targets may be searched among the enzymes preventing the degradation of the BCR-ABL protein. The data on the specific inhibition of deubiquitinase USP1 activity in vitro in K562 cells have been presented. A vast array of other targetable enzymes interacting with the BCR-ABL protein and affecting its stability and activity remains an extensive field for further study. A putative role of protein phosphatase 2A in this context is discussed.

**Keywords:** chronic myeloid therapy, BCR-ABL, differentiation therapy, stemness phenotype, USP1 deubiquitinase, K562 cells

## 1. Introduction

Chronic myeloid leukemia (CML) is a clonal hematopoietic stem cell (HSC) disorder characterized by a reciprocal translocation (t(9;22)(q34;q11)) resulting in a *BCR-ABL1* fusion gene and the chimeric p210 BCR-ABL1 protein possessing constitutive kinase activity [1, 2]. The specific inhibitors of tyrosine kinase activity (TKI), such as imatinib, have found deserved recognition in the frontline therapy of CML [3]. Nevertheless, acquired therapy resistance represents a serious problem,



IntechOpen

preventing long-term remission in CML patients despite advances in the development of more potent TKIs [4]. Meanwhile, various mechanisms are involved in the development of resistance to therapy that are not completely dependent on BCR-ABL1 activity [5]. Therefore, the search for alternative therapies, including differentiation therapy, is currently in the limelight. Over the past years, the inadequacy of many CML therapies has been shown to result from their failure to target LSCs. The control over the differentiation of CML LSCs may represent a useful therapeutic approach [6]. In fact, various agents, including growth factors, cytokines, chemical substances, etc., have been identified as differentiating agents for CML cells in vitro. Nevertheless, the mechanisms mediating the differentiation effects may be diverse, affecting different regulatory pathways in leukemic cells. The analysis of the signaling pathways and their components as targets of the induced differentiation of CML cells is an important step in developing novel therapeutic strategies in the context of cell differentiation therapy. Here, we present our recent data on the expression of the genes involved in the differentiation of CML cells and the genes coding for stemness biomarkers in K562 cells exposed to alpha-tocopherol as a putative agent capable of contributing to CML cell differentiation.

Actually, several alternative and complementary approaches for CML treatments are currently underway in the hope of overcoming resistance to TKI, as well as identifying different pathways and molecular targets that prevent uncontrolled proliferation of leukemic blast cells in CML. Such strategies are directed not at the inhibition of the constitutively activated tyrosine kinase but rather at the degradation of this chimeric protein and the eventual elimination of cells from the pathological clone [7]. Although various modalities of BCR-ABL1 degradation are being developed and tested in in vitro systems, the lack of sufficient specificity is still a problem to be solved. Targeting deubiquitinating enzymes may provide an alternative strategy for the selective modulation of BCR-ABL1 protein levels in CML cells, which has proven to be effective in in vitro studies [8]. The data on the use of specific inhibitors of the deubiquitinase USP1 activity in vitro in K562 cells will be discussed.

The future prospects of the research should be based on the analysis of the proteins interacting with BCR-ABL in hematopoietic stem cells and leukemic blasts [9]. Some challenging novel strategies, such as the specific reactivation of protein phosphatase 2A (PP2A), have been proposed [10]. The recent literature data on the interplay between the activity of BCR-ABL1 and PP2A in CML cells and the putative ways to modulate PP2A activity will be disclosed in the context of further studies of PP2A-reactivating modalities. Moreover, the recent literature data on the interplay between the activity of BCR-ABL1 and PP2A in CML cells and the putative ways to modulate PP2A activity suggest that alpha-tocopherol is among the known PP2A-reactivating molecules.

## 2. Alpha-tocopherol and G-CSF change the expression of genes associated with the differentiation of K562 CML cells while downregulating EMT-associated stemness biomarkers

Myeloid master regulator transcription factor CCAAT/enhancer-binding protein alpha (C/EBPα) is considered as a major molecular trigger of myelopoiesis, however, CML blast cells lose their differentiation potential and acquire uncontrolled proliferation [11]. Down-regulation of C/EBPα is correlated with the progression of CML to blast crisis, while the restoration of C/EBPα expression in the BCR-ABL + cell line by TKI results in terminal granulocytic differentiation [12]. These findings, along with many others, suggest that C/EBPα could be considered a putative target in differentiation therapies for myeloid leukemias, including CML.

Historically, a variety of chemical agents were found to be able to induce differentiation of CML cells in vitro, many of them being rather toxic and not intended for any practical purposes [13]. Meanwhile, it has long been known that some of the hematopoietic leukemia cell lines of myeloid origin, such as K562 or CML blasts, may be induced to differentiate by various cytokines [14].

In our previous chapter in the IntechOpen monograph [15], we presented data on the putative role of alpha-tocopherol in the targeted induction of the myeloid master regulator transcription factor C/EBPα in K562 cells. Earlier, we also demonstrated the ability of alpha-tocopherol to restore C/EBPα expression, resulting in C/EBPα-mediated expression of the gene for the G-CSF receptor (*CSF3R*) in K562 cells [16]. Meanwhile, G-CSF-R is expressed not only on myeloid cells such as neutrophils but also on HSCs and progenitor cells [17]. Taken together, these facts suggest a functional interrelationship between C/EBPα, G-CSF-R, and G-CSF [18, 19].

The possible involvement of G-CSF in the differentiation of CML blast cells has not yet been studied in detail. The loss of G-CSF and G-CSFR is a characteristic feature associated with the arrested differentiation of CML blast cells. G-CSF is currently used in CML patients, improving responsiveness to TKI therapy. It is known that normal myelopoiesis in bone marrow is supported by G-CSF, which is constitutively produced by bone-forming osteoblasts [20–22]. Meanwhile, tissue non-specific (liver/bone/kidney) alkaline phosphatase (TNAP), representing an osteogenic differentiation regulator of osteoblasts, seems to be important in supporting the HSC niche in bone marrow [23]. G-CSF and TNAP can be suggested as mutually dependent markers of HSC differentiation. Moreover, TNAP, encoded by the *ALPL* gene, is detectable in differentiated neutrophils and monocytes and is induced by G-CSF treatment [24].

Previously, we have shown that in K562 CML cells, the *ALPL* gene was not expressed, while the expression of the aberrant isoform of alkaline phosphatase, namely leukemic stem cell-associated placental-like alkaline phosphatase (PLAP), was observed [15, 25]. This aberrant isoform of alkaline phosphatase is considered potentially useful as a tumor-associated marker [26]. Moreover, according to our data, alpha-tocopherol is effective in restoring the expression of C/EBPα and TNAP in K562 cells, both being tightly associated with the possible reactivation of myeloid differentiation potential [25].

In the present study, we further explored the differentiation potential of alpha-tocopherol and G-CSF by analyzing the expression of *CEBPB* and *ALPL* genes, which encode factors critical for myeloid differentiation, versus the expression of genes encoding leukemic stemness-associated transcription factors SNAIL and OCT4 in K562 CML cells.

K562 cells were treated for 72 hours either with alpha-tocopherol acetate at a dose of 100 μM (300 mg/mL stock solution; Lekchim, Ukraine) or G-CSF (Filstim, Biofarma, Ukraine) at a dose of 1 μg/mL (10,000 IU). A real-time RT-PCR was performed using the following primers (**Table 1**). The gene expression was quantified using the 2Δ-Ct method with normalization to *GAPDH* mRNA expression.

| Gene | Forward primer | Reverse primer |
|---|---|---|
| *ALPL* | 5′-TGGCCGGAAATACATGTACCC-3′ | 5′-TTCCGTGCGGTTCCAGATG-3′ |
| *ALPP* | 5′-AAGGGCAGAAGAAGGACAAA | 5′-GTCGTGTTGCACTGGTTAAAG |
| *CEBPB* | 5′-CAA GAA CAG CAA CGA GTA CCG-3′ | 5′-GTC ACT GGT CAA CTC CAG CAC-3′ |
| *CDH1* | 5′-TGCCCAGAAAATGAAAAAGG-3′ | 5′-GTGTATGTGGCAATGCGTTC-3′ |
| *SNAI1* | 5′-CAGACCCACTCAGATGTCAA-3′ | 5′-CATAGTTAGTCACACCTCGT-3′ |
| *POU5F1* | 5′-GCACTGTACTCCTCGGTCCCTTTCCC-3′ | 5′-CTTCCCTCCAACCAGTTGCCCCAAAC-3′ |
| *GAPDH* | 5′-CGCTCTCTGCTCCTCCTGTT-3′ | 5′-CCATGGTGTCTGAGCGATGT-3′ |

**Table 1.**
*Primers used in the study.*

Our findings demonstrate that either alpha-tocopherol or G-CSF upregulated *CEBPB* expression, but alpha-tocopherol caused 2.54 times higher upregulation of the gene compared to G-CSF (**Figure 1A**). Both single agents also upregulated *ALPL* expression to the same extent (**Figure 1B**). Coincidentally, with the expression of factors affecting differentiation of myeloid cells, we observed a significant increase in the expression of the *CDH1* gene (E-cadherin) (**Figure 1C**).

Although E-cadherin is not associated directly with the differentiation of myeloid cells, the treatment of K562 cells with a differentiating agent such as phorbol ether results in an increasing expression of E-cadherin [27]. Such upregulation of the *CDH1* gene, coinciding with the increasing expression of markers of myeloid differentiation such as C/EBP and TNAP induced by alpha-tocopherol or G-CSF, prompted us to analyze the expression of several transcription factors that are usually upregulated in the setting of the loss of E-cadherin. It is known that the activation of transcription factors such as SNAIL, SLUG, TWIST1, ZEB1, ZEB2, and several others, which bind to E-box sequences in the *CDH1* gene promoter, negatively regulates E-cadherin expression [28]. Moreover, these factors have been found to be associated with the maintenance of cell pluripotency and stemness in hematological malignancies [29].

While EMT has been implicated in promoting the stemness of cancer cells, which is important for tumorigenesis and metastasis in solid tumors, the role of EMT and the major transcription factors involved in this process in the case of hematopoietic malignancies remains to be elucidated. Several studies have assumed a role for such EMT-related factors as SNAIL, TWIST, and others in the pathogenesis of myeloid malignancies [30, 31].

We found a significant down-regulation of *SNAI1, ALPP*, and *POU5F1* expression in K562 cells incubated with alpha-tocopherol or G-CSF. Alpha-tocopherol was as effective as G-CSF in decreasing *ALPP* and *POU5F1* RNA expression, while its effect on *SNAI1* expression was less noticeable compared to G-CSF (**Figure 2**).

Earlier, we have already found PLAP expression in peripheral blood cells of patients with CML in blast crisis, acute myeloid leukemia, and polycythemia vera, as well as in K562 cells [25]. In this study, we showed that PLAP downregulation is triggered not only by alpha-tocopherol but also by G-CSF as a specific inducer of myeloid differentiation. Moreover, the changes in the expression of PLAP caused by the differentiation agents are paralleled by the downregulation of the transcription factors SNAIL and OCT4 which are associated with the maintenance of CSC stemness.

DOI: http://dx.doi.org/10.5772/intechopen.1013747

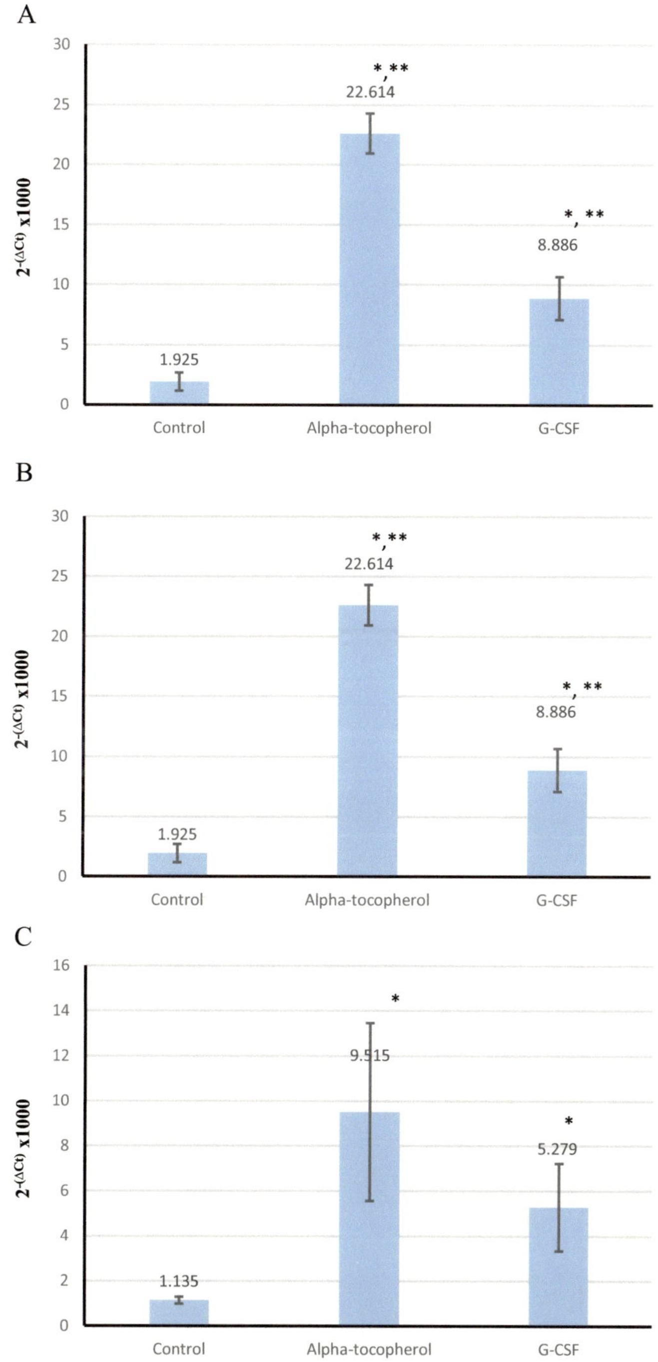


**Figure 1.**

*The relative mRNA expression levels of the* CEBPB *(A),* ALPL *(B), and* CDH1 *(C) genes. K562 cells were incubated either with alpha-tocopherol acetate at a dose of 100 μM (300 mg/mL stock solution; Lekchim, Ukraine) or G-CSF (Filstim, Biofarma, Ukraine) at a dose of 1 μg/mL (10,000 IU) for 72 h. Total RNA was extracted and converted to cDNA using Qiagen's QuantiTect Rev. Transcription Kit (Qiagen, Germany). A real-time RT-PCR was performed using the SYBR Green protocol. All the experiments were conducted in triplicate. The gene expression was quantified using the* $2^{-\Delta Ct}$ *method with normalization to GAPDH mRNA expression.* * $p < 0.01$ *compared to control cells;* ** $p < 0.01$ *between the effects of alpha-tocopherol and G-CSF treatments.*

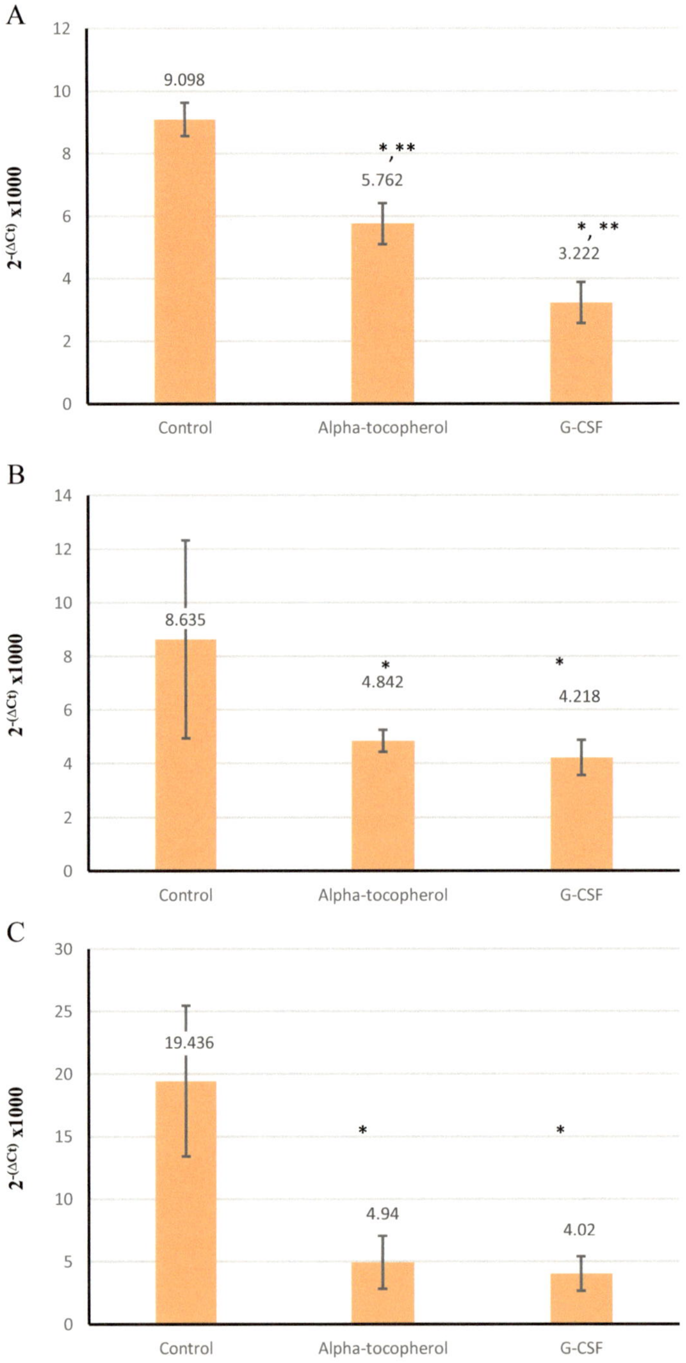


**Figure 2.**

*The relative mRNA expression levels of* SNAI1 (A), ALPP (B), *and* POU5F1 (C) *genes. K562 cells were incubated either with alpha-tocopherol acetate at a dose of 100 µM (300 mg/mL stock solution; Lekchim, Ukraine) or G-CSF (Filstim, Biofarma, Ukraine) at a dose of 1 µg/mL (10,000 IU) for 72 h. Total RNA was extracted and converted to cDNA using Qiagen's QuantiTect Rev. Transcription Kit (Qiagen, Germany). A real-time RT-PCR was performed using the SYBR Green protocol. All the experiments were conducted in triplicate. The gene expression was quantified using the $2^{-\Delta Ct}$ method with normalization to GAPDH mRNA expression.* * $p < 0.01$ (A, C) *or* $p < 0.05$ (B) *compared to control cells;* ** $p < 0.01$ *between the effects of alpha-tocopherol and G-CSF treatments.*

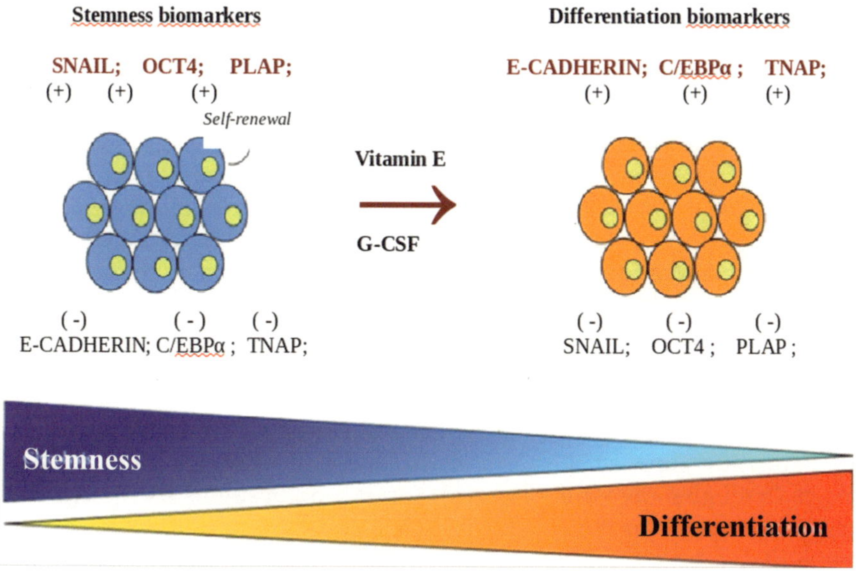


**Figure 3.**
*Schematic diagram of the stimulated differentiation potential in CML blast cells by alpha-tocopherol and G-CSF. The repression of the stemness biomarkers SNAIL, OKT4, and PLAP results in the activation of the differentiation biomarkers E-cadherin, C/EBPα, and TNAP. Alpha-tocopherol decreases stemness markers expression with accompanying increase in differentiation potential. The diagram illustrates the reciprocal relations between stemness phenotype of stem-like blast cells and their differentiation potential with the balance between the transcription factors involved in cell differentiation and cell stemness.*

Taken together, the results obtained have emphasized that the detected in vitro downregulation of the stemness biomarkers SNAIL, PLAP, and OKT4 at the RNA level in K562 CML cells, induced by alpha-tocopherol or G-CSF exposure, is accompanied by the activation of the expression of the differentiation biomarkers E-cadherin, C/EBPα, and TNAP. This suggests a complementary approach to CML therapy using agents that change the balance between the transcription factors involved in cell differentiation, on the one hand, and cell stemness, on the other hand, as part of differentiation therapy for myeloid leukemias. This is summarized schematically in **Figure 3,** illustrating the reciprocal relations between the leukemic pluripotent stemness phenotype and the differentiation potential of leukemic stem-like blast cells in CML myeloid differentiation, outlining the future strategies for differentiation therapy of CML.

## 3. USP1-targeted therapy as a novel strategy for chronic myeloid leukemia

While TKI therapy remains a mainstream approach in the treatment of CML in the chronic phase, the development of treatment resistance necessitates the search for novel strategies that involve numerous targets in cells other than BCR-ABL1 itself. Meanwhile, one of the major challenges in modern oncology is the pharmacological inaccessibility of many oncoproteins, primarily due to the absence of well-defined ligand-binding pockets or specific molecular targets.

Deubiquitinating enzymes (DUBs) provide an alternative strategy for the selective modulation of oncoprotein levels, as DUBs remove ubiquitin moieties from protein substrates, thereby regulating their stability, functional activity, and involvement in diverse cellular processes. DUBs play a pivotal role in maintaining cellular homeostasis by controlling a broad spectrum of essential functions, including the preservation of genomic integrity, regulation of gene expression, stem cell proliferation and differentiation, cell cycle progression, chromosome segregation during mitosis, and signal transduction pathways, particularly those mediated by growth factors. Alterations in their expression or enzymatic activity disrupt cellular equilibrium, ultimately contributing to the onset and progression of various pathological states, such as neurodegenerative disorders, immune system dysfunctions, and malignant neoplasms [32–34].

DUB inhibition may restore sensitivity to cytotoxic agents, a factor of particular importance for aggressive and recurrent cancer forms. Incorporating DUB inhibitors into therapeutic regimens holds the potential to enhance the efficacy of conventional chemo and radiotherapy. This synergistic interaction positions DUB-targeted strategies as a promising component of the next generation of anticancer therapies [35].

The role of several DUBs as putative targets for CML therapy has been demonstrated in various in vitro studies. In particular, DUBs are shown to be associated with the BCR-ABL1 signaling pathway, and the suppression of these enzymes may be an effective way to induce BCR-ABL1 ubiquitination and degradation [36, 37]. Thus, for example, the use of an inhibitor of USP9X results in BCR-ABL1 ubiquitination followed by the apoptosis of both TKI-sensitive and resistant CML cells [38]. Numerous data provide evidence that targeting DABs, in particular, USP7, USP9X, USP10, USP15, USP25, and USP47, can effectively overcome TKIs resistance in CML, which may represent a novel strategy for CML treatment [39].

Among approximately 100 DUBs, ubiquitin-specific protease 1 (USP1) stands out as one of the most extensively studied members. USP1 has emerged as a promising therapeutic target for various cancer types. Several inhibitors of USP1 slow down the growth of leukemic cell lines, including CML [40]. In our previous studies, we demonstrated that USP1 forms a protein complex with BCR-ABL1, a key driver of CML pathogenesis. Immunofluorescence analysis, followed by confocal microscopy, revealed that this protein complex localizes within the nuclei of CML cells [41]. The discovery of the USP1–BCR-ABL interaction prompted an investigation into the phosphorylation status of USP1. To this end, the phosphorylated USP1 isoforms were examined through immunoprecipitation of tyrosine-phosphorylated proteins, followed by immunofluorescence analysis in K562 cells, to assess their subcellular distribution. These experiments confirmed the presence of USP1 phosphorylated on tyrosine residues in CML cells [42]. Notably, the USP1 isoforms most prominently represented were those interacting with BCR-ABL1. Tyrosine-phosphorylated proteins were predominantly localized at the cell periphery, which likely reflects the high kinase activity of BCR-ABL1, as a substantial fraction of this oncoprotein also accumulates in these regions. Based on these findings, we hypothesize that BCR-ABL1 phosphorylates the deubiquitinase USP1, enhancing its catalytic activity. This post-translational modification may alter the balance of ubiquitination and deubiquitination processes, contributing to the disruption of cellular homeostasis and supporting leukemogenic signaling [8, 41, 42].

By deubiquitinating specific substrate proteins, USP1 plays a critical role in their stabilization, which is of particular interest for the development of novel therapeutic strategies in CML. In our study, we found that inhibition of USP1 deubiquitinating activity by a highly selective inhibitor, ML323 used in concentrations of 52 nM and 76 nM, resulted in a marked reduction of BCR-ABL1 levels in CML cells. A noticeable decrease in BCR-ABL1 levels was observed as early as 1.5 hours after ML323 administration, and the maximal effect was achieved in 3 hours. After 6 hours of exposure, BCR-ABL1 levels began to rise and returned to near-control levels by 12 hours (**Figure 4**). We hypothesize that this rebound may be attributed to either a loss of ML323 inhibitory activity or compensatory reactivation of USP1 via alternative mechanisms unaffected by the compound. Another plausible factor could be proteasomal overload, characterized by the impaired degradation of an abnormally large pool of misfolded proteins. This phenomenon, while extensively described in neurodegenerative diseases, remains insufficiently explored in cancer, despite the fact that malignantly transformed cells are characterized by elevated protein synthesis rates and significant accumulation of misfolded proteins [41, 43, 44].

The immunofluorescence analysis further revealed that ML323 treatment substantially reduced the colocalization of BCR-ABL and USP1, with the lowest levels detected at 1.5 h and 3 h of incubation, coinciding with the time points of minimal BCR-ABL1 abundance in cells [44].

Based on the results obtained, we believe that USP1 removes ubiquitin from the oncoprotein BCR-ABL1, thereby preventing its proteasomal degradation, which leads to its accumulation and subsequent disease progression. Therefore, USP1 could be considered a promising therapeutic target in CML. Lowering BCR-ABL levels through activation of cellular degradation systems represents a novel therapeutic approach for CML that does not depend on the mutational variability of ABL kinase domains and enables highly selective modulation of oncoprotein abundance, opening new avenues for USP1-targeted CML therapy.

It is also worth mentioning that, apart from the use of selective inhibitors of the DABs, one of the promising directions in developing targeted CML therapy involving the ubiquitin-proteasome system is represented by constructing bifunctional

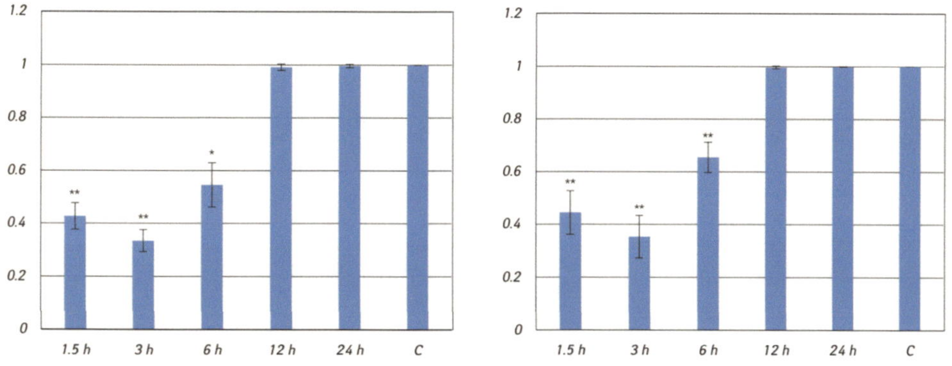


**Figure 4.**
*Effects of ML323 — low-molecular-weight USP1 inhibitor — on BCR-ABL protein level after 24-h incubation with 52 nM (A) or 76 nM (B) ML323. The normalized values of band areas in Western blot of the lysates of CML K562 cells treated with ML323 are presented. Anti-BCR-ABL antibody (1:1000; MA1-153, Thermo Fisher Scientific, USA) was used for detection. The effect of ML323 was reversible, and in 12 h, the BCR-ABL level returned to the control values.* * $p < 0.01$, ** $p < 0.001$ *as compared to controls.*

inhibitors that simultaneously target the BCR-ABL1 molecule and recruit E3 ubiquitin ligase [45]. Therefore, specific degradation of BCR-ABL1 may be achieved in several alternative ways.

## 4. Protein phosphatase 2A (PP2A) as an important node in kinase–phosphatase homeostasis and a presumable therapeutic target in CML

The prospective therapeutic modalities for CML targeted at BCR-ABL1 should consider various networks guiding the balance between the synthesis and degradation of this tyrosine kinase and the interactions of this oncoprotein with dozens of other molecules. One such molecule is protein phosphatase 2A (PP2A), which possesses tumor suppressor function [46]. This serine/threonine-specific phosphatase plays a key role in the regulation of multiple signaling pathways that control cell proliferation, differentiation, and apoptosis. PP2A exists as a heterotrimeric holoenzyme that includes three subunits: A (structural), B (regulatory), and C (catalytic) [47] (**Figure 5**)

PP2A functions primarily as a heterotrimer composed of a scaffold A (PPP2R1A/PPP2R1B), a catalytic C (PPP2CA/PPP2CB), and one of multiple regulatory B subunits (B/B55/PR55; B′/B56/PR61; B″/PR72/PPP2R3; B‴/striatin family/STRN). The combinatorial pairing of A/C with the numerous B-subunits yields more than 100 distinct holoenzymes, providing substrate specificity and directing PP2A to nuclear, cytoplasmic, or membrane-proximal locales [48]. The PP2A-A and PP2A-C exist in the form of a dimeric complex – core enzyme, while the regulatory B subunit exists as a single unit. The combination of the

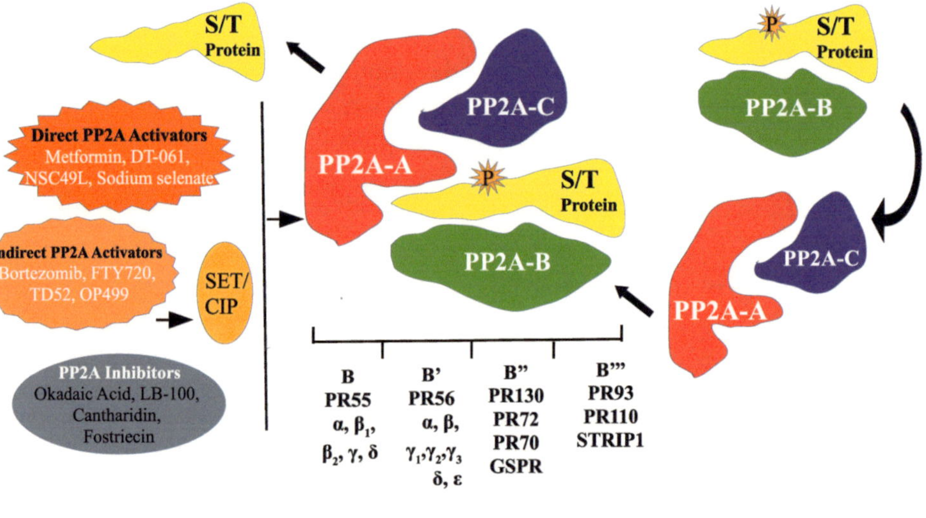


**Figure 5.**

*Schematic representation of the formation of holoenzyme PP2A from subunits and modulators affecting the enzyme action. Each heterotrimeric PP2A holoenzyme consists of heterodimeric core enzyme, comprising a scaffolding subunit (A) and a catalytic subunit (C), and a variable regulatory subunit (B). Serine/threonine (S/T) phosphorylated (P) proteins interact with substrate-specific regulatory subunit (B), which subsequently recruits the substrate protein to the core enzyme. Holoenzyme formation is stabilized by the binding of the phosphorylated substrate to B subunit. The subunit C then dephosphorylates the substrate. The direct and indirect PP2A activators as well as PP2A inhibitors affecting the activity of PP2A are depicted.*

dimer and trimer results in the formation of an active holoenzyme. PP2A thereby governs Wnt, mTOR, PI3K–AKT, and MAPK signaling, and regulates G1→S transition, DNA synthesis, and mitotic entry.

PP2A acts as a tumor suppressor, limiting the activity of oncogenic signaling cascades, including PI3K/AKT, MAPK, and JAK/STAT. PP2A inactivation is observed in many hematologic tumors and is associated with mutations, expression of endogenous inhibitors (e.g., SET), or interaction with oncoproteins [49]. In CML, BCR-ABL1 promotes PP2A inactivation via the activation of the SET inhibitor, which enhances oncogenic signaling [50]. It should be noted that A and C subunits are usually expressed unchanged in CML, and the suppression of PP2A activity is entirely determined by a significant decrease in B56α and partially in B55α subunits. B56α primarily affects the signaling pathways Wnt and p53, and B55α affects the pathways related to the mitotic cycle and metabolism (CDK1, Akt) [51, 52]. Detailing these interactions will further identify a specific subunit of PP2A complex as a possible therapeutic target. The restoration of PP2A activity leads to the suppression of clonal CML cells, including TKI-resistant ones.

Besides CML, in Ph-positive AML, the role of PP2A is also critical. Inactivation of the enzyme is associated with disruption of cell cycle control and increased proliferative potential. Experimental data indicate that activation of PP2A can lead to remission in preclinical models [53].

Therefore, the restoration of PP2A activity is considered a promising strategy for the treatment of CML and AML. The PP2A activators include FTY720 (fingolimod), OP449, DT-061, and small molecules that stabilize the holoenzyme [54, 55]. On the other hand, PP2A inhibitors, such as okadaic acid and cantharidin, are used in experimental studies to investigate the biological functions of the enzyme [56].

It is intriguing that PP2A in CML cells may be reactivated by targeting various molecules rather than PP2A itself. Among such targets, one can mention JAK [57]. The suppression of SET (PP2A inhibitor) in CML cells also brings about PP2A reactivation [58]. O'Connor et al. [59] stated that several different strategies aimed at PP2A reactivation may exist, namely inhibition of endogenous inhibitors of PP2A, targeted disruption of posttranslational modifications on PP2A subunits, and direct targeting of PP2A.

Combination approach to therapy seems to be the most optimal. Bringing the main first-line drug to the forefront, and based on this, possible practical recommendations for their use can be proposed. Foremost, priority should be given to identify the particular B-subunits expressed and involved in the disease setting (e.g., B56α vs. B56 δ vs. B55α), since their substrate specificity and localization may differ substantially. Finally, the rational combination should be tailored. Because PP2A intersects with Wnt/mTOR/PI3K–AKT/MAPK, PP2A modulators may be combined with the appropriate kinase inhibitors or DNA-damaging agents, using biomarkers to avoid inactivation of tumor suppressor holoenzymes.

PP2A is at the center of cellular signaling homeostasis. Its heterotrimeric, B-subunit–directed organization explains both its reach and its tractability: by learning which holoenzymes are pathologically silenced (e.g., via SET or CIP2A) and which pathways they police, one can reactivate the right PP2A complexes or – in select contexts – transiently inhibit them to amplify therapeutic efficacy. This strategy is rapidly becoming actionable as better holoenzyme-selective chemical tools and robust methylation/B-subunit biomarkers emerge. Further research in this area is necessary to design clinically applicable drugs [59, 60].

## 5. Conclusion

While the introduction of TKIs into clinical practice turned out to be a revolution in CML treatment, being at the frontline of CML therapy for several decades, the acquired resistance to the therapy has become a growing source of concern. This brings to the forefront the development of novel treatment strategies and complementary therapies that may be helpful in overcoming treatment resistance, especially during the phase of the blast crisis. These novel approaches envisage the in-depth study of the BCR-ABL1 signaling pathways and the molecules interacting with this constitutively active tyrosine kinase. The differentiation therapy, proven as a valuable tool in the treatment of some types of cancer, may also be useful for CML treatment. It is of practical interest that several biologically active molecules, such as alpha-tocopherol, are as effective in vitro as G-CSF in upregulating the expression of factors associated with granulocyte differentiation. We demonstrated that the upregulation of the expression of the myeloid master regulator transcription factor C/EBPα, induced in CML cells by alpha-tocopherol or G-CSF, is accompanied by the downregulation of the stemness-related factors SNAIL, PLAP, and OKT4. The further search for applicable inducers of differentiation in CML cells should take into account that such substances may affect the balance between the transcription factors involved in cell differentiation and the factors involved in the maintenance of cell stemness.

Several methods that could be useful in CML therapy are focused not on the inhibition of the activity of the uncontrollably expressed BCR-ABL1 in CML cells but on the increased degradation of this tyrosine kinase, which finally leads to the decreased burden of the oncoprotein in the leukemic cells. Among such novel strategies are the methods targeting DUBs and PP2A since these enzymes are components of two major regulatory pathways determining the turnover of proteins and their activity. The challenging task in the practical development of these approaches is the search for the corresponding inhibitors possessing increased specificity, as well as the identification of the most appropriate components of the ubiquitin-proteasome system and the specific subunits of the PP2A system to serve as specific targets directed toward BCR-ABL1. Finally, combination therapy will open new prospects in CML treatment.

## Author details

Lyudmyla P. Shvachko[1*], Svitlana Antonenko[1], Michael Zavelevich[2], Irene Gartovska[3], Mykhailo Dybkov[1], Dmytro Gur`yanov[1] and Gennadii Telegeev[1]

1 Institute of Molecular Biology and Genetics, the National Academy of Sciences of Ukraine, Kyiv, Ukraine

2 R.E. Kavetsky Institute of Experimental Pathology, Oncology and Radiobiology, the National Academy of Sciences of Ukraine, Kyiv, Ukraine

3 Kyiv Regional Oncology Center, Center for Hematology and Bone Marrow Transplantation, Kyiv, Ukraine

*Address all correspondence to: l.shvachko@ukr.net

## References

[1] Shtivelman E, Lifshitz B, Gale RP, et al. Fused transcript of abl and bcr genes in chronic myelogenous leukaemia. Nature. 1985;**315**(6020):550–554. DOI: 10.1038/315550a0

[2] Quintàs-Cardama A, Cortes J. Molecular biology of bcr-abl1-positive chronic myeloid leukemia. Blood. 2009;**113**:1619–1630. DOI: 10.1182/blood-2008-03-144790

[3] Pophali PA, Patnaik MM. The role of new tyrosine kinase inhibitors in chronic myeloid leukemia. Cancer Journal. 2016;**22**(1):40–50. DOI: 10.1097/PPO.0000000000000165

[4] Jabbour E, Parikh SA, Kantarjian H, et al. Chronic myeloid leukemia: Mechanisms of resistance and treatment. Hematology/Oncology Clinics of North America. 2011;**25**(5):981–995. DOI: 10.1016/j.hoc.2011.09.004

[5] Hamilton A, Helgason GV, Schemionek M, et al. Chronic myeloid leukemia stem cells are not dependent on BCR-ABL kinase activity for their survival. Blood. 2012;**2119**: 1501–1510

[6] Mojtahedi H, Yazdanpanah N, Rezaiel N. Chronic myeloid leukemia stem cells: Targeting therapeutic implications. Stem Cell Research & Therapy. 2021;**12**:603. DOI: 10.1186/s13287-021-02659-1

[7] Cruz-Rodriguez N, Deininger MW. Novel treatment strategies for chronic myeloid leukemia. Blood. 2025;**145**(9):931–943. DOI: 10.1182/blood.2024026312

[8] Antonenko S, Zavelevich M, Telegeev G. The role of USP1 deubiquitinase in the pathogenesis and therapy of cancer. Acta Biochimica Polonica. 2023;**70**(2):219–231. DOI: 10.18388/abp.2020_6636

[9] Miroshnychenko D, Dubrovska A, Maliuta S, Telegeev G, Aspenström P. Novel role of pleckstrin homology domain of the BCR-ABL protein: Analysis of protein-protein and protein-lipid interactions. Experimental Cell Research. 2010;**316**(4):530–542. DOI: 10.1016/j.yexcr.2009.11.014

[10] Goswami S, Mani R, Nunes J, et al. PP2A is a therapeutically targetable driver of cell fate decisions via a c-Myc/p21 axis in human and murine acute myeloid leukemia. Blood. 2022;**139**(9):1340–1358. DOI: 10.1182/blood.2020010344

[11] Porse BT, Bryder D, Theilgaard-Mönch K, et al. Loss of C/EBP alpha cell cycle control increases myeloid progenitor proliferation and transforms the neutrophil granulocyte lineage. Journal of Experimental Medicine. 2005;**202**(1):85–96. DOI: 10.1084/jem.20050067

[12] Pulikkan JA, Tenen DG, Behre G. C/EBPα deregulation as a paradigm for leukemogenesis. Leukemia. 2017;**31**(11):2279–2285. DOI: 10.1038/leu.2017.229

[13] Bianchi N, Ongaro F, Chiarabelli C, Gualandi L, Mischiati C, Bergamini P, Gambari R. Induction of erythroid differentiation of human K562 cells by cisplatin analogs. Biochemical Pharmacology. 2000;**60**(1):31–40. DOI: 10.1016/s0006-2952(00)00297-5

[14] Leung KN, Mak NK, Fung MC. Cytokines in the differentiation therapy of leukemia: From laboratory investigations to clinical applications. Critical Reviews in Clinical Laboratory Sciences. 2005;**42**:473–514. DOI: 10.1080/10408360500295154

[15] Shvachko L, Zavelevich M, Gluzman D, Telegeev G. Vitamin E in Chronic Myeloid Leukemia (CML) Prevention. In: P Erkekoglu, J Scherer Santos, editors. Vitamin E in Health and Disease - Interactions, Diseases and Health Aspects. London: IntechOpen; 2021. DOI: 10.5772/intechopen.96452

[16] Shvachko LP, Zavelevich MP, Gluzman DF, Telegeev GD. Vitamin E induces transcription factor C/EBP alpha and G-CSFR in K562 cells. Experimental Oncology. 2018;**40** (4):328–331

[17] McKinstry WJ, Li CL, Rasko JE, et al. Cytokine receptor expression on hematopoietic stem and progenitor cells. Blood. 1997;**89**:65–71

[18] Semerad GL, Liu F, Gregory AD, et al. G-CSF is an essential regulator of neutrophil trafficking from the bone marrow to the blood. Immunity. 2002;**17**(4):413–423. DOI: 10.1016/s1074-7613(02)00424-7

[19] Greenbaum AM, Link DC. Mechanisms of G-CSF-mediated hematopoietic stem and progenitor mobilization. Leukemia. 2011;**25** (2):211–217. DOI: 10.1038/leu.2010.248

[20] Calvi LM, Adams GB, Weibrecht KW, et al. Osteoblastic cells regulate the haematopoietic stem cell niche. Nature. 2003;**425**(6960):841–846. DOI: 10.1038/nature02040

[21] Taichman RS, Emerson SG. Human osteoblasts support hematopoiesis through the production of granulocyte colony-stimulating factor. Journal of Experimental Medicine. 1994;**179**: 1677–1682. DOI: 10.1084/jem.179.5.1677

[22] Fulzele K, Krause DS, Panaroni C, et al. Myelopoiesis is regulated by osteocytes through Gs -dependent signaling. Blood. 2013;**121**(6):930–939. DOI: 10.1182/blood-2012-06-437160

[23] Nakamura T, Nakamura-Takashi A, Kasahara M, et al. Tissue-nonspecific alkaline phosphatase promotes the osteogenic differentiation of osteoprogenitor cells. Biochemical and Biophysical Research Communications. 2020;**524**(3):702–709. DOI: 10.1016/j.bbrc.2020.01.136

[24] Udristioiu A, Iliescu RG, Cojocaru M, Joanta A. Alkaline phosphatase isoenzymes and leukocyte alkaline phosphatase score in patients with acute and chronic disease: A brief review. British Journal of Medicine & Medical Research. 2014;**4**(1):340–350. DOI: 10.9734/BJMMR/2014/3309

[25] Shvachko LP, Zavelevich MP, Gluzman DF, Telegeev GD. Aberrant expression of placental-like alkaline phosphatase (PLAP) in chronic leukemia cells in vitro and its modulation by vitamin E. Experimental Oncology. 2020;**42**(1):1–4. DOI: 10.32471/exp-oncology.2312-8852.vol-42-no-1.14285

[26] Su Y, Zhang X, Bidlingmaier S, et al. ALPPL2 is a highly specific and targetable tumor cell surface antigen. Cancer Research. 2020;**80**(20): 4552–4564. DOI: 10.1158/0008-5472.CAN-20-1418

[27] Zhou ZL, Ma J, Tong MH, et al. Nanomechanical measurement of adhesion and migration of leukemia cells with phorbol 12-myristate 13-acetate treatment. International Journal of Nanomedicine. 2016;**11**: 6533–6545

[28] Dongre A, Weinberg RA. New insights into the mechanisms of epithelial-mesenchymal transition and implications for cancer. Nature Reviews Molecular Cell Biology. 2019; **20**(2):69–84. DOI: 10.1038/s41580-018-0080-4

[29] Chen SC, Liao TT, Yang MH. Emerging roles of epithelial-mesenchymal transition in hematological malignancies. Journal of Biomedical Sciences. 2018;**25**:37. DOI: 10.1186/s12929-018-0440-6

[30] Carmichael CL, Wang J, Nguyen T, et al. The EMT modulator SNAI1 contributes to AML pathogenesis via its interaction with LSD1. Blood. 2020;**136** (8):957–973. DOI: 10.1182/blood.2019002548

[31] Dong CY, Liu XY, Wang N, et al. Twist-1, a novel regulator of hematopoietic stem cell self-renewal and myeloid lineage development. Stem Cells. 2014;**32**(12):3173–3182. DOI: 10.1002/stem.1803

[32] Tu R, Ma J, Zhang P, et al. The emerging role of deubiquitylating enzymes as therapeutic targets in cancer metabolism. Cancer Cell International. 2022;**22**(1):130. DOI: 10.1186/s12935-022-02524-y

[33] Mullard M, Lavaud M, Regnier L, et al. Ubiquitin-specific proteases as therapeutic targets in paediatric primary bone tumours? Biochemical Pharmacology. 2021;**194**:114797

[34] Liu J, Leung CT, Liang L, et al. Deubiquitinases in cancers: Aspects of proliferation, metastasis, and apoptosis. Cancers. 2022;**14**(14):3547. DOI: 10.3390/cancers14143547

[35] Jin S-K, Baek K-H. Unraveling the role of deubiquitinating enzymes on cisplatin resistance in several cancers. Biochimica Et Biophysica Acta. Reviews on Cancer. 2025;**1880**(2):189297. DOI: 10.1016/j.bbcan.2025.189297

[36] Jiang S, Wang X, He Y, et al. Suppression of USP7 induces BCR-ABL degradation and chronic myelogenous leukemia cell apoptosis. Cell Death & Disease. 2021;**12**(5):456. DOI: 10.1038/s41419-021-03732-6

[37] Shibata N, Ohoka N, Tsuji G, et al. Deubiquitylase USP25 prevents degradation of BCR-ABL protein and ensures proliferation of Ph-positive leukemia cells. Oncogene. 2020;**39** (19):3867–3878. DOI: 10.1038/s41388-020-1253-0

[38] Sun H, Kapuria V, Peterson LF, et al. BCR-ABL ubiquitination and USP9x inhibition block kinase signaling and promote CML cell apoptosis. Blood. 2011;**117**(11):3151–3162. DOI: 10.1182/blood-2010-03-276477

[39] Lei H, Wang J, Hu J, et al. Deubiquitinases in hematological malignancies. Biomarker Research. 2021;**9**:66

[40] Mistry H, Hsieh G, Buhrlage SJ, et al. Small-molecule inhibitors of USP1 target ID1 degradation in leukemic cells. Molecular Cancer Therapeutics. 2013;**12** (12):2651–2662. DOI: 10.1158/1535-7163.MCT-13-0103-T

[41] Antonenko S, Gurianov D, Telegeev G. Colocalization of USP1 and

PH domain of BCR-ABL oncoprotein in terms of chronic myeloid leukemia cell rearrangements. Cytology & Genetics. 2016;**50**(5):352–356

[42] Antonenko S, Polishchuk Y, Telegeev G. Phosphorylation of Tyr sites of USP1 protein in K562 cells as a factor in chronic myeloid leukemia progression. The Bulletin of Ukrainian Society of Geneticists and Breeders [Visnik Ukrains'kogo Tovaristva Genetikiv I Selekcioneriv]. 2019;**17** (2):145–149. DOI: 10.7124/visnyk. utgis.17.2.1214

[43] Antonenko S, Kravchuk I, Telegeev G. Interaction of BCL-ABL oncoprotein with the GLG1 protein in K562 cells: Its role in the pathogenesis of chronic myeloid leukemia. Cytology & Genetics. 2020;**54**(1):48–54

[44] Antonenko S, Telegeev G. Inhibition of USP1, a new partner of BCR-ABL, results in decrease of BCR-ABL level in K562 cells. Experimental Oncology. 2023;**42** (2):109–114. DOI: 10.32471/exp-oncology.2312-8852.vol-42-no-2.14533

[45] Cruz-Rodriguez N, Tang H, Bateman B, et al. BCR::ABL1 Proteolysis-targeting chimeras (PROTACs): The new frontier in the treatment of Ph+ leukemias? Leukemia. 2024;**38**:1885–1893

[46] Perrotti D, Neviani P. Protein phosphatase 2A (PP2A), a druggable tumor suppressor in Ph1(+) leukemias. Cancer and Metastasis Reviews. 2008;**27** (2):159–168

[47] Sents W, Ivanova E, Lambrecht C, Haesen D, Janssens V. The biogenesis of active protein phosphatase 2A holoenzymes: A tightly regulated process creating phosphatase specificity. The FEBS Journal. 2013;**280** (2):644–661. DOI: 10.1111/j.1742-4658. 2012.08579.x

[48] Xu Y, Xing Y, Chen Y, et al. Structure of the protein phosphatase 2A holoenzyme. Cell. 2006;**127**(6):1239–1251. DOI: 10.1016/j.cell.2006.11.033

[49] Cristóbal I, Garcia-Orti L, Cirauqui C, et al. PP2A impaired activity is a common event in acute myeloid leukemia and its activation by forskolin has a potent anti-leukemic effect. Leukemia. 2011;**25**(4):606–614. DOI: 10.1038/leu.2010.294

[50] Neviani P, Harb JG, Oaks JJ, et al. PP2A-activating drugs selectively eradicate TKI-resistant chronic myeloid leukemic stem cells. The Journal of Clinical Investigations. 2013;**123**: 4144–4157

[51] Peris I, Romero-Murillo S, Vicente C, et al. Regulation and role of the PP2A-B56 holoenzyme family in cancer. Biochimica Et Biophysica Acta. Reviews on Cancer. 2023;**1878** (5):188953. DOI: 10.1016/j. bbcan.2023.188953

[52] Fowle H, Zhao Z, Xu Q, et al. PP2A/B55α substrate recruitment as defined by the retinoblastoma-related protein p107. Elife. 2021;**10**:e63181

[53] Oaks JJ, Santhanam R, Walker CJ, et al. Antagonistic activities of the immunomodulator and PP2A-activating drug FTY720 (Fingolimod) in Jak2-driven hematologic malignancies. Blood. 2013;**122**(11):1923–1934. DOI: 10.1182/blood-2013-03-492181

[54] Sangodkar J, Farrington CC, McClinch K, et al. All roads lead to PP2A: Exploiting the therapeutic potential of this phosphatase. The FEBS

Journal. 2016;**283**(6):1004–1024. DOI: 10.1111/febs.13573

[55] Leonard D, Huang W, Izadmehr S, et al. Selective PP2A enhancement through biased heterotrimer stabilization. Cell. 2020;**181**(3):688–701. DOI: 10.1016/j.cell.2020.03.038

[56] Li M, Guo H, Damuni Z. Purification and characterization of two potent heat-stable protein inhibitors of protein phosphatase 2A from bovine kidney. Biochemistry. 1995;**34**(6):1988–1996. DOI: 10.1021/bi00006a020

[57] Gallipoli P, Cook A, Rhodes S, et al. JAK2/STAT5 inhibition by nilotinib with ruxolitinib contributes to the elimination of CML CD34+ cells in vitro and in vivo. Blood. 2014;**124**:1492–1501

[58] Agarwal A, MacKenzie RJ, Pippa R, et al. Antagonism of SET using OP449 enhances the efficacy of tyrosine kinase inhibitors and overcomes drug resistance in myeloid leukemia. Clinical Cancer Research. 2014;**20**:2092–2103

[59] O'Connor CM, Perl A, Leonard D, et al. Therapeutic targeting of PP2A. The International Journal of Biochemistry & Cell Biology. 2018;**96**:182–193

[60] Ruvolo PP. The broken 'off' switch in cancer signaling: PP2A as a regulator of tumorigenesis, drug resistance, and immune surveillance. BBA Clinical. 2016;**6**:87–99. DOI: 10.1016/j.bbacli. 2016.08.002

Chapter 6

# Treatment Modifications Due to Toxicities During Chemotherapy in Leukemia

*Dao-Hai Cheng and Wen-Ling Chen*

## Abstract

Leukemia poses serious threats to human health among adults and children, and combination chemotherapy is widely used to treat the acute forms of the disease. However, the toxicity of chemotherapy remains a concern, as it is a common cause of treatment modifications – delay or interruption, dose reduction, drug substitution, or even omission of specific medications – throughout the treatment period. Here, we provide an overview of treatment modifications due to chemotherapy-induced toxicities in leukemia. Literature on PubMed and Google Scholar was searched using relevant keywords up to March 2025. Overall, toxicity-induced treatment modifications were common during chemotherapy in leukemia, with frequency varying across patients, regimens, and disease subtypes. Despite some conflicting results, the limited data available in the literature suggest that treatment delays during intensive phases are associated with inferior survival outcomes or an increased risk of relapse. Toxicity-induced treatment modifications remain a concern during chemotherapy in acute leukemia. Given its potential impact on clinical outcomes, further attention should be paid to this issue throughout the course of treatment in the future.

**Keywords:** chemotherapy, leukemia, toxicity, treatment, modification, delay

## 1. Introduction

Hematological malignancies are myeloid and lymphoid neoplasms that can affect the bone marrow, blood cells, and lymphatic system. They are estimated to account for 6.5% of all cancer cases worldwide, with around 9% in economically developed regions such as the United States and Europe [1]. The age-standardized incidence rate of hematological malignancies globally is estimated at 17 per 100,000 individuals, with over 700,000 deaths annually [2]. Hematological malignancies comprise a diverse group of neoplastic disorders that can be broadly categorized into four basic types based on the cell of origin, clinical behavior, and primary anatomical site of involvement: leukemia, multiple myeloma, non-Hodgkin lymphoma (NHL), and Hodgkin lymphoma (HL). Out of these categories, leukemia can further be classified into four main subtypes according to the cell lineage from which they arise and the speed of disease progression: acute lymphoblastic leukemia (ALL), acute myeloid leukemia (AML), chronic lymphocytic leukemia (CLL), and chronic myeloid leukemia (CML), among which ALL is the most common cancer during childhood, while AML, CLL, and CML primarily affect adults.

With the advancement in understanding of disease pathogenesis and the application of contemporary treatment approaches and supportive measures, remarkable progress in clinical outcomes has been achieved over the past several decades for hematologic malignancies, such as childhood ALL [2], HL [3], and certain subsets of AML (e.g., acute promyelocytic leukemia [APL], core-binding factor AML) [4], a unique subtype of AML. Nevertheless, treatment outcomes for hematologic malignancies in lower-income regions are less impressive compared to developed countries [5]. In addition, there are distinct differences in overall prognosis among disease subtypes or patient populations. For instance, while the long-term survival and cure rate of ALL in children, especially in low-risk patients, currently exceed 90% when using front-line therapeutic approaches [6], the outcomes for children with high-risk disease are relatively disappointing compared to the results achieved in low-risk subjects, with five-year overall survival (OS) ranging from 50% to 70%[5]. Furthermore, the prognosis for ALL or AML in elderly adults remains poor, with less than 20%–50% achieving five-year OS [7, 8]. Thus, there remains a need for more effective strategies to improve the treatment outcomes of patients with hematologic malignancies.

There are a number of therapeutic options available for the treatment of patients with leukemia, including systemic combination chemotherapy, immunotherapy, molecular targeted therapy, and sometimes stem cell transplantation or radiation therapy [9]. Selection of a treatment regimen for specific patients is individualized based on the clinical features of the patients (age, performance status, and concomitant comorbidities), morphological appearances of the disease, such as subtypes (ALL, AML, CLL, and CML), risk groups (low-risk, intermediate-risk, and high-risk), and disease stages (newly diagnosed, in remission, and refractory or recurrent) that the patients are at. Personal choice, cost considerations, and drug availability may also influence this choice.

During the treatment of leukemia, a number of factors can influence whether predetermined criteria established in the protocols can be strictly adhered to. These factors may include varied access to health services or drugs, the presence of treatment-related toxicities or medical events, the existence of comorbid conditions, the compliance of health professionals or patients with protocols or guidelines, and the regional socioeconomic level (e.g., financial condition, insurance status). Consequently, in clinical practice, delays in scheduled therapy, reductions in dose intensity, premature termination of treatment, and substitution or even omission of specific chemotherapy agents in subsequent phases may be required.

It is generally considered that maintaining treatment intensity is one of the determinants of clinical outcomes in patients with leukemia. However, treatment-related toxicities can increase with the enhancement of chemotherapy. Toxicity-induced modification of treatment, possibly leading to lower dose intensity and potentially compromising treatment outcomes, is a common source of anxiety for health care professionals, patients, and/or their guardians.

In view of the role of chemotherapy in the treatment of leukemia, toxicity associated with chemotherapy remains a concern, as it is a common factor leading to dose reduction, temporary interruption, treatment delay, discontinuation of therapy, or switching to alternative drugs throughout the treatment period. In this chapter, we provide an overview of toxicity-induced modifications of treatment during chemotherapy in patients with leukemia. Literature searches were conducted in PubMed and Google Scholar for relevant articles, limited to the English language, using appropriate keywords up to March 2025. This review specifically focuses on conventional chemotherapy, and targeted therapeutic agents (e.g., immunotherapies or molecularly targeted drugs) are beyond the scope of this article and thus will not be discussed here.

## 2. Overview of toxicity-induced treatment modifications during chemotherapy in leukemia

Combination chemotherapy is the cornerstone for the treatment of acute leukemia (see **Table 1**). Throughout the course of treatment, patients often experience a wide variety of side effects, including hematological [10, 11] and non-hematological events [12–14], which not only impair the patient's quality of life and increase the cost of treatment but may also lead to treatment modifications (e.g., dose reduction, temporary interruption, drug substitution, or therapy discontinuation), potentially affecting the patient's prognosis [15, 16]. There is wide variability in the frequency of dose adjustments across patients, regimens, and malignancy types, potentially due to differences in the regimens administered, patient characteristics, supportive care measures adopted per institution, and analytical methods used (e.g., based on patients or cycles, criteria for definition of the dose-adjustment indicators).

### 2.1 Acute lymphoblastic leukemia

Although various novel treatment options (e.g., targeted therapies, chimeric antigen receptor T-cell (CAR-T) therapy, and other immunotherapies) are available, conventional intensive chemotherapy remains the main treatment approach for ALL, primarily based on the synergy of several effective chemotherapeutic drugs.

Treatment for ALL can generally be classified into induction, consolidation, intensification, and maintenance phases [6], although protocols may vary across clinical trials, patient populations, or geographic regions. Induction (remission induction), the first phase of treatment, aims to reduce disease burden and restore normal hematopoiesis to achieve complete remission. Treatment in remission induction is usually based on combination chemotherapy that may include vincristine, glucocorticoids (e.g., prednisone, dexamethasone), anthracyclines (e.g., daunorubicin, doxorubicin), L-asparaginase, and cyclophosphamide [6]. Intrathecal (IT) chemotherapy is often used as a strategy for central nervous system (CNS) prophylaxis and treatment. Consolidation, also called postremission or intensive therapy, is a phase of treatment to eliminate residual leukemic cells potentially remaining after achieving remission. The treatment approach used in this phase is based on risk status and comprises four to six cycles of short-term, relatively intensive combination chemotherapy every two weeks, usually involving agents with different mechanisms of action, such as cytarabine (Ara-C), high-dose methotrexate (MTX) ($>500\ mg/m^2$), vincristine, L-asparaginase, 6-mercaptopurine (6-MP), and glucocorticoids [6]. IT chemotherapy is typically continued at this stage. Intensification (reinduction) uses drugs similar to those used in induction

| Leukemia | Treatment phase or disease stage | Typical treatment regimen | Overall treatment modifications during chemotherapy |
|---|---|---|---|
| ALL | Induction | Regimen typically comprising vincristine, glucocorticoids (e.g., prednisone, dexamethasone), and anthracyclines (e.g., daunorubicin, doxorubicin); other chemotherapy drugs, such as L-asparaginase or cyclophosphamide, may also be added; intrathecal chemotherapy | A substantial proportion (e.g., 50%–90%) of patients underwent treatment modifications (dose reductions, delays, and omissions) during the intensive phases due to toxicities [5, 17–21]. Despite some inconsistent or conflicting results [21–23], the limited data available in the literature suggest that treatment delays [18–20, 24–26] or substantial changes in treatment regimens due to severe toxicities [5, 27, 28] are associated with inferior survival outcomes or an increased risk of relapse |
| | Consolidation | Several cycles of combination chemotherapy every two weeks, usually including Ara-C, high-dose MTX, vincristine, L-asparaginase, 6-MP, and glucocorticoids; intrathecal chemotherapy | |
| | Intensification | Use drugs similar to those used in induction therapy | |
| | Maintenance | Daily oral 6-MP and weekly oral low-dose MTX, with or without pulses of vincristine and glucocorticoids (e.g., dexamethasone), intrathecal chemotherapy | 40%–90% of patients experienced treatment interruptions or therapy delays during the maintenance phase, and there was a tendency for fewer relapses in patients who had longer delays [19, 21, 29] |
| AML | Induction | "7 + 3" regimen: the combination of Ara-C for seven days and a three-day course of an anthracycline (e.g., daunorubicin, idarubicin), with or without targeted therapy agents; intrathecal Ara-C or MTX may be used to treat CNS leukemia | 0%–2% of patients discontinued treatment due to death or toxicity in standard induction regimens [30] |
| | Consolidation | Treatment with several cycles of more dose-intensive Ara-C-based regimens; intrathecal chemotherapy | Toxicities cause longer durations of hospitalization, withdrawal from further consolidation cycles (15% due to infection or persisting cytopenia), or even treatment-related deaths (5%–7% of patients); less than 60% of the patients completed all four planned cycles of chemotherapy [31, 32] |
| | Maintenance | Maintenance therapy with targeted agents (e.g., FLT3 inhibitors) or oral azacitidine | Temporary treatment interruptions, dose reductions, and permanent discontinuations due to toxicities were noted in 43%, 16%, and 13% of AML patients receiving oral azacitidine therapy [33] |
| CLL | Symptomatic progression | With the introduction of highly effective targeted agents, traditional chemotherapy is less commonly used; the FCR regimen (fludarabine, cyclophosphamide, and rituximab) may be indicated for patients with mutated IGHV | Dose modifications (e.g., reductions, delays, or omissions) were applied to 75% of patients due to toxicity or organ function [34]; 40%–75% of the patients completed all six cycles of FCR therapy [34, 35] |

| Leukemia | Treatment phase or disease stage | Typical treatment regimen | Overall treatment modifications during chemotherapy |
|---|---|---|---|
| CML | Whole phases | Treatment mainly involves targeted therapies (e.g., TKIs) and allogeneic HSCT; conventional cytotoxic drugs (i.e., non-TKI anti-CML agents) are less commonly used but may be considered in certain circumstances | Temporary treatment interruption, dose reduction, and discontinuation of therapy occurred in 50%, 25%–30%, and 7%–10% of patients receiving chemotherapy-based regimens, respectively [36, 37, 56] |

*Abbreviations: ALL, acute lymphoblastic leukemia; AML, acute myeloid leukemia; CLL, chronic lymphocytic leukemia; IGHV, immunoglobulin heavy-chain variable region gene; CML, chronic myeloid leukemia; TKI, tyrosine kinase inhibitor; MTX, methotrexate; Ara-C, cytarabine; 6-MP, 6-mercaptopurine; FLT3, FMS-like tyrosine kinase 3; EFS, event-free survival; OS, overall survival.*

**Table 1.**
*Typical treatment regimens and overall toxicity-induced treatment modifications during chemotherapy in leukemia.*

therapy. Maintenance is delivered for two to three years following reinduction, with the aim of preventing disease relapse after consolidation and reinduction therapy. Treatment for ALL in the maintenance phase typically comprises a lower intensity of antimetabolite therapy, such as daily oral 6-MP and weekly oral low-dose MTX, with or without periodic administration of vincristine-glucocorticoid pulses. IT treatment with MTX continues during the maintenance phase.

Patients receiving ALL treatment are often burdened with a wide range of toxicities that may impair quality of life and cause longer lengths of stay, higher readmission rates, or even worse survival [12, 39]. In addition to causing approximately 1%–3% of deaths in pediatric ALL patients and possibly a higher frequency in adults [40, 41], severe toxicity often leads to various forms of treatment modifications, such as early discontinuation of therapy, schedule delays, drug substitution, and dose reduction in subsequent cycles. Based on a retrospective analysis of toxicity registration from children treated with the NOPHO ALL-2008 protocol, more than half of the patients (37/73) underwent treatment modifications due to toxicities, among which 59% (22/37), 24% (9/37), and 16% (6/37) were dose omission or reduction, treatment delay, and delay combined with dose modification, respectively [17]. The most common toxicities causing treatment modifications in the cohort were vincristine-induced peripheral neuropathy and asparaginase-associated toxicities (e.g., anaphylaxis and allergy, acute pancreatitis, and thrombosis). Skeletal complications (e.g., osteonecrosis) and CNS toxicities (e.g., MTX-related stroke-like syndrome) were less frequently reported as reasons for treatment modifications during chemotherapy. Toxicity-induced modifications appear to be more frequent in low- and middle-income countries. During the chemotherapy period for pediatric ALL across four South American centers, treatment delays of greater that two weeks occurred in 56% of patients, with 63% and 47% of these delays attributed to infections and other drug-related toxicities, respectively [5]. Modifications to treatment regimens (e.g., dose omission, discontinuation of asparaginase or MTX) were also present throughout all phases of therapy. In pediatric patients with ALL or lymphoblastic lymphoma during the COVID-19 pandemic, chemotherapy interruptions occurred in up to 87% of patients in response to toxicities and COVID-19 [42].

Although the definition of treatment delay varies across studies, a substantial proportion (e.g., 50%–90%) of patients has been reported to experience some delay (see **Table 2**). The effect of treatment delay on clinical prognosis has been investigated in a number of studies. In a large prospective study conducted by Kumar et al. [18], delays in postremission intensification therapy were observed in 99.5% (1071/1076) of the patients and negatively affected survival outcomes (e.g., OS or event-free survival (EFS)) in those receiving allografting or nontransplant therapy. A similar association between treatment delay during the intensive phase (induction or consolidation) and clinical outcomes was reported in several other studies [19, 20, 24–26]. However, a lack of effect [21, 22] or even a beneficial effect [23] of treatment delay on clinical prognosis (relapse or survival) has also been described during the intensive phases. Despite this, it should be noted that substantial changes in treatment regimens due to severe toxicities could be associated with inferior survival outcomes, as evidenced by significantly lower three-year EFS (51.4% vs. 73.2%) and OS (65.6% vs. 81.1%) in patients with substantial changes to the original treatment regimen [5], or demonstrated by markedly reduced relapse-free survival (RFS) (2.9 vs. 4.7 years; $p < 0.001$) and OS (3.2 vs. 4.9 years; $p < 0.001$) in patients experiencing extreme treatment-related toxicities requiring significant therapy modification [27].

Regarding treatment delay during maintenance, according to the study by de Oliveira et al. [29], 84% of pediatric patients (61/73) experienced chemotherapy interruptions due to bone marrow or liver toxicity. Patients with chemotherapy interruptions for a period exceeding 2% of the total duration of the maintenance phase had a significantly higher probability of EFS (80.3% vs. 33.3%) and a 4.9-fold lower risk of relapse than those with interruptions below 2% ($p = 0.0001$ and $p = 0.001$, respectively) [29]. Similar results were observed by Yeoh et al. [21], who reported that longer treatment delays during maintenance were associated with a trend toward fewer relapses, with a significant difference observed between the lowest and highest quartiles. However, in the study by Agrawal et al. [19], treatment delays in maintenance therapy were not found to affect survival outcomes (e.g., EFS, RFS, and OS).

To reduce treatment-related morbidity and mortality while maintaining efficacy, researchers have sought proactively to refine therapy regimens, including modifications in chemotherapeutic drug doses, timing of administration, duration of therapy, and combination with other effective agents. For example, as a front-line pediatric ALL protocol, St. Jude Total Therapy has evolved greatly over the past 60 years, during which many modifications (e.g., reduction in or removal of more toxic treatments such as VP16 or CNS irradiation in certain patients) were introduced to improve OS and maintain safety [43]. For adult patients with ALL, using a reduced dose of pegaspargase (≤1,000, median 500 IU/($m^2$ dose)) as part of the pediatric-inspired induction regimen (CALGB 10,403), the total grade 3/4 toxicity observed during induction was lower than with the standard dose (>1,000, median 2,500 IU/($m^2$ dose)), while the majority of patients (84.6%, 22/26) receiving the reduced dose still achieved therapeutic asparaginase activity levels [44]. In infants with ALL, treatment approaches have changed continuously over the past three decades, which include modifications in chemotherapy regimens such as lowering doses of drugs (e.g., daunorubicin), substitution with less toxic agents (e.g., replacement of native asparaginase with pegaspargase), or omission of specific chemotherapy agents (e.g., cyclophosphamide) during induction [45, 46].

| Patient | Disease | Age (years) | No. of patients | Country or region | Study design | Treatment protocol or method | Delay measurement or definition | Incidence of delay | Reasons or risk factors for delay | Impact of delay on prognosis | Reference |
|---|---|---|---|---|---|---|---|---|---|---|---|
| Adults | Ph − ALL | 20–65 | 1,076 | International | Prospective | ECOG 2993/ MRC UK ALLXII | Number of days beyond the scheduled initiation date of postremission intensification therapy | 99.5% of the patients experienced a delay | Increasing age, being Black, female sex, being Asian, and experiencing significant toxicities during the induction phase | Delays negatively affected survival outcomes in patients receiving allografting or nontransplant therapy | [18] |
| Children and adults | ALL | 1–57 | 149 | India | Retrospective | MCP-841, GMALL and BFM-95 | Duration from the start of a particular phase to the initiation of the next phase of treatment exceeds the predetermined criteria | Delay during induction, consolidation, and maintenance: 52%, 65%, and 42%, respectively | Contributors to delay in the induction phase: age group of ≤14 years; causes for delay in the intensive or maintenance phase: neutropenia, thrombocytopenia, liver toxicity, and patient noncompliance | Treatment delays in the intensive phase were linked to inferior EFS and RFS; delays in maintenance therapy did not affect survival outcomes | [19] |
| Children | ALL | Median (IQR): 5 (2.73–10.39) | 127 | Poland | Retrospective | ALLIC BFM 2002 and 2009 protocols | Delay at any milestone time point (Day 8, Day 15, and Day 33) during the induction phase | Delays occurred in 66% cases | Disease complications, treatment-related toxicities, or weekend delay | Delays at specific time points increased the risk of relapse or death in HR patients | [20] |
| Children | ALL | Mean: 6.5 | 141 | Australia | Retrospective | Study 8, COG, and Study 9 | Cumulative length of delays in the entire chemotherapy, intensive, or maintenance phase exceeding seven days | 94.7% of all patients experienced some delay | Low blood counts, severe infections other than bacteremia, and febrile neutropenia | Longer treatment delays did not affect relapse risk during the entire treatment or intensive phase, but they were associated with a reduced risk of relapse during the maintenance phase | [21] |
| Children | ALL | 1.1–18.9 | 227 | Australia | Retrospective | ANZCCSG ALL Study-V and Study-VI | Delay at three early time points: end of induction, midconsolidation, and end of consolidation | Delay in starting consolidation attributable to low ANC or platelet count: 2% | Myelotoxicity (low ANC or platelet count) | Delay at any measured time point was not associated with the risk of subsequent relapse | [22] |

| Patient | Disease | Age (years) | No. of patients | Country or region | Study design | Treatment protocol or method | Delay measurement or definition | Incidence of delay | Reasons or risk factors for delay | Impact of delay on prognosis | Reference |
|---|---|---|---|---|---|---|---|---|---|---|---|
| Children | ALL | < 16 | 287 | China | Retrospective | CCLG-ALL -2008 | Cumulative delay between treatment courses beyond seven days is considered a delay | Cumulative delay greater than seven days: 77% | Myelosuppression, septicemia, pulmonary infection, drug-induced liver injury, severe mucositis, infectious diseases, pancreatitis, and complications | Cumulative delay greater than four weeks was an independent prognostic factor for relapse | [24] |
| Adults | AML and ALL | 18–71 | AML: 61; ALL: 31 | China | Retrospective | Induction followed by consolidation chemotherapy | Interval days during intensive chemotherapy | Mean interval ≥30 days: 76% | Grade IV toxicity, concomitant underlying diseases | Mean interval ≥50 days during intensive therapy was an independent negative factor for OS and PFS | [25] |
| Children | ALL | < 18 | 242 | Turkey | Retrospective | Modified BFM 90 and BFM-TR ALL 2000 protocols | Number of days beyond phase duration or phase transition during therapy | Total delay >11 days: 80% | Febrile neutropenia, hepatosteatosis, drug toxicity, electrolyte/metabolite disturbances, hemophagocytosis, and neurologic events | Patients with a total delay of more than 11 days had better OS and EFS than those with shorter periods of interruption | [23] |
| Children | ALL | 1–16 | 99 | Colombia | Prospective | Historic cohort: a modified BFM regimen; study population: LLA-ACHOP 2006 | Time of delay in the initiation of the PIII block of therapy | ≥4 weeks of delay: 63% | Complications of therapy (e.g., infections) and non-medical reasons (e.g., delayed insurance approval, lack of beds or appointments, and other non-medical causes) | Delayed initiation of the PIII block of therapy (≥4 weeks) predicted markedly inferior DFS | [26] |
| Children | ALL | 1.3–16.3 | 73 | Brazil | Retrospective | GBTLI-93 | Duration of interruption of chemotherapy during the maintenance phase | Inappropriate interruptions: 37%; appropriate interruptions: 84% | Inappropriate interruptions due to non-adherence to the treatment protocol or appropriate interruptions because of significant toxicities | Patients with longer appropriate suspensions during maintenance had a higher probability of EFS and a lower risk of relapse | [29] |
| Children | ALL | 1–21 | 537 | USA | Retrospective | Intensive chemotherapy followed by maintenance treatment | Days of delay to the start of maintenance therapy | Most patients had some delay | Treatment-related complications, older mean age, higher intensity regimen, Hispanic or Black ethnicity, and T-ALL | Treatment delays before the start of maintenance therapy do not impact survival, but patients with extreme toxicities have significantly inferior RFS and OS | [27] |

| Patient | Disease | Age (years) | No. of patients | Country or region | Study design | Treatment protocol or method | Delay measurement or definition | Incidence of delay | Reasons or risk factors for delay | Impact of delay on prognosis | Reference |
|---|---|---|---|---|---|---|---|---|---|---|---|
| Children | ALL | < 18 | 752 | Four countries in South America | Retrospective | Institutional regimen | Treatment held >2 weeks | Delay >2 weeks: 56.0% | Infection, other toxicities, and resource constraints (e.g., drug shortages or bed unavailability) | Patients with a treatment delay of more than two weeks had more relapses but fewer deaths, and consequently, longer OS | [5] |

*Abbreviations: ALL, acute lymphoblastic leukemia; AML, acute myeloid leukemia; EFS, event-free survival; RFS, relapse-free survival; DFS, disease-free survival; OS, overall survival; PFS, progression-free survival; IQR, interquartile range; ANC, absolute neutrophil count; HR, high-risk.*

**Table 2.**
*Main studies on toxicity-induced treatment delays during chemotherapy in leukemia.*

## 2.2 Acute myeloid leukemia

The treatment of patients with AML is based on whether the disease is newly diagnosed or recurrent. Chemotherapy for newly diagnosed AML can be divided into remission induction and consolidation (also called postremission) therapy. The backbone of chemotherapy for remission induction is anthracycline and Ara-C-based therapy, most commonly as the "7 + 3" regimen, using the combination of Ara-C for seven days and a three-day course of an anthracycline (e.g., daunorubicin, idarubicin), with or without targeted therapy agents [47]. Consolidation therapy for AML patients in remission is usually based on regimens consisting of different doses of Ara-C [48]. Maintenance therapy is less commonly included in many current treatment protocols and clinical trials, but therapy with targeted agents (e.g., FLT3 inhibitors) or oral azacitidine may improve outcomes [49]. For refractory or recurrent AML, intensive salvage chemotherapy or reduced-intensity therapy, including targeted therapy, can be considered. IT Ara-C or MTX may be used to treat CNS leukemia.

During the induction phase, approximately 3%–9% of patients discontinued treatment due to death or toxicity when using the standard regimen ("7 + 3" or high-dose Ara-C + idarubicin, IA) [30]. Toxicities associated with consolidation therapy for patients with AML mainly manifest as febrile neutropenia, gastrointestinal complications (nausea and vomiting, oral mucositis, and diarrhea), and neurotoxicity, which can cause longer durations of hospitalization, withdrawal from further consolidation cycles, or even treatment-related deaths [31, 32]. In the maintenance treatment of oral azacitidine therapy, temporary treatment interruptions, dose reductions, and permanent discontinuation due to adverse events (AEs) were noted in 43%, 16%, and 13% of AML patients, respectively. The most common AEs leading to dosing modifications were severe myelosuppression, high-grade gastrointestinal toxicity, and other AEs [33].

## 2.3 Chronic lymphocytic leukemia

Given the indolent nature of the disease, treatment is not indicated for asymptomatic or minimally affected patients with CLL, and clinical observation is generally considered the standard of care [50]. However, for patients who are experiencing symptomatic or progressive CLL, treatment is usually required. With the introduction of highly effective targeted agents such as covalent Bruton tyrosine kinase (BTK) inhibitors, B-cell leukemia/lymphoma 2 (BCL2) inhibitors, and monoclonal anti-CD20 antibodies, conventional chemotherapy is less commonly used. Purine analogs (e.g., fludarabine) and alkylating agents (e.g., cyclophosphamide, bendamustine, chlorambucil) are used in conjunction with monoclonal antibodies as chemoimmunotherapy for CLL. Chemoimmunotherapy with several cycles of the FCR regimen (fludarabine, cyclophosphamide, and rituximab) may be considered as a treatment option for patients with mutated IGHV [51].

Although effective for CLL, the FCR regimen can also cause a variety of AEs (e.g., myelosuppression, gastrointestinal toxicity, infusion-related reactions, and skin rash), and treatment modifications may be required in severe cases [34, 52]. According to the study by Hillmen et al. [34], 54%, 14%, and 12% of CLL patients receiving the chemoimmunotherapy regimen of FCR developed grade ≥3 leukopenia, anemia, and sepsis during the first year after treatment, respectively, and dose modifications (e.g., reductions, delays, and omissions) were applied based on toxicity and organ function in 75% of patients throughout treatment. The occurrence of toxicity may also lead to some patients being unable to complete all planned therapy. In a survey evaluating outcomes after FCR therapy in CLL patients from five centers in Spain, less than half of the patients completed all six cycles of FCR therapy, with the main reasons for discontinuation being cytopenia and infection [35].

### 2.4 Chronic myeloid leukemia

CML is traditionally classified into three phases: chronic phase (CP), accelerated phase (AP), and blast phase (BP). The most commonly used agents for CML therapy nowadays are different generations of BCR-ABL1 tyrosine kinase inhibitors (TKIs) [53]. Non-TKI drugs (hydroxyurea, omacetaxine, interferon, hypomethylating agents, and others) are less commonly used but may be considered in certain circumstances. For example, hydroxyurea is used in symptomatic patients to reduce white blood cell counts and shrink enlarged spleens. Omacetaxine may be administered to patients with refractory CML or intolerance to TKI therapies. For patients with CML-BP or those not responding to TKIs, treatment options are rather limited, and the prognosis is generally poor. Although there is no complete consensus, intensive chemotherapy or a less toxic regimen may be used as induction therapy or as a conditioning regimen before allogeneic hematopoietic stem cell transplantation (HSCT) for such patients [54–56]. IT chemotherapy is considered for prophylaxis or treatment of CNS involvement.

Toxicities can be severe during induction chemotherapy, and treatment modifications may be required. Using a time-sequenced regimen consisting of a purine analog (fludarabine or cladribine) plus high-dose Ara-C and an anthracycline (idarubicin or mitoxantrone), or a "7 + 3" regimen (standard-dose Ara-C plus an anthracycline (idarubicin or daunorubicin)) as induction chemotherapy (both plus a TKI) for patients with CML-BP myeloid phenotype, a substantial number of patients experienced febrile neutropenia (100%) or at least one grade ≥ 3 non-hematologic toxicity (66.7%) [57]. A higher incidence of toxicity was also observed when dasatinib and decitabine were used in combination in patients with advanced CML, which led to temporary treatment interruption, dose reduction, and discontinuation of therapy in 50%, 27%, and 10% of patients, respectively [36]. Similarly, when using combination therapy with imatinib and low-dose decitabine, more than a quarter of patients with CML-AP or myeloid CML-BP had a reduced dose of decitabine in the second or later treatment cycle due to prolonged myelosuppression [37]. In patients with lymphoid CML-BP who were treated with Hyper-CVAD (cyclophosphamide, vincristine, doxorubicin, dexamethasone, alternating with MTX and Ara-C) plus a TKI (imatinib or dasatinib), high rates of grade 3–4 hematological toxicity (100%) and infections (59%) were recorded, with 7% and 9% of patients discontinuing treatment, respectively [38].

With regards to the conditioning regimen, there is wide variability in the dosing of chemotherapy and the agents employed. In general, a higher-intensity regimen is associated with more toxic effects and less relapse. Adopting a personalized conditioning regimen to achieve an appropriate balance between efficacy and safety (specifically non-hematological toxicities) is critical for patients receiving HSCT [58]. To reduce the toxicity of conditioning regimens, the introduction of reduced-intensity conditioning, less toxic agents (e.g., replacement of busulfan with treosulfan), or control of serum concentrations through therapeutic drug monitoring (TDM) may be considered [59].

## 3. Toxicity-induced treatment modifications for commonly used chemotherapeutic agents in leukemia

The treatment of many hematologic malignancies is grounded in a broad spectrum of effective chemotherapeutic agents, such as asparaginase, antimetabolites (e.g., MTX, Ara-C, thiopurines), anthracyclines, vinca alkaloids (e.g., vincristine, vindesine, vinblastine), alkylating agents, and corticosteroids. **Table 3** outlines toxicity-induced treatment modifications for commonly used chemotherapeutic agents in leukemia.

### 3.1 Asparaginase

Administration of multiple doses of asparaginase is an important component of a multi-agent chemotherapeutic regimen for the treatment of ALL in pediatric and young adult patients. Asparaginase has a distinctive toxicity profile, including hypersensitivity, pancreatitis, thrombosis, hepatotoxicity, and encephalopathy [74]. Although the majority of asparaginase-related AEs are reversible, manageable, and nonfatal [75], there are still some toxicities that require modifications of drug therapy. According to the study by Duffy et al. [5], asparaginase-related toxicities requiring intermittent dose omission or permanent discontinuation were observed in approximately one-fifth of pediatric ALL patients. For mild-to-moderate laboratory abnormalities (e.g., ≤Grade 2 transaminitis, hyperbilirubinemia, hyperglycemia, hyperlipidemia) that are commonly observed in chemotherapy, asparaginase therapy is usually not discontinued or delayed [75]. Certain high-grade asparaginase toxicities, including hypertriglyceridemia, hyperglycemia, and thrombosis, can be managed with symptomatic or supportive measures; in this situation, asparaginase therapy may also be continued in subsequent cycles without dose reduction. For instance, continuation of asparaginase therapy is recommended with the concomitant use of low-molecular-weight-heparin anticoagulation therapy for patients with thrombosis [60]; asparaginase can be continued if blood glucose returns to the normal range when treated with insulin in severe hyperglycemia cases [75]. For patients at high risk for hypertriglyceridemia, asparaginase treatment can be continued with careful monitoring, and severe hypertriglyceridemia may resolve with appropriate management (e.g., hydration, low-fat diet, and pharmacological interventions) without requiring an interruption or modification in treatment [76].

The common asparaginase-related toxicities that may lead to dose modification or schedule delay include clinical pancreatitis, high-grade hepatotoxicity, hypersensitivity reactions, and serious thrombotic or hemorrhagic events. In a recent study conducted by Ishida et al., asparaginase discontinuation was reported in 8.9% (16/179) and 14.3% (19/133) of pediatric patients with T-ALL and T-lymphoblastic lymphoma, respectively, and the most common reasons for discontinuation of asparaginase were pancreatitis, thrombosis, and allergy [28]. Importantly, the effect

| Chemotherapy drug | Toxicity | Potential treatment modification associated with toxicity | Reference |
|---|---|---|---|
| Asparaginase | ≥Grade 3 hypersensitivity to asparaginase or pegaspargase | Discontinue and switch to *Erwinia* asparaginase | [60–62] |
| | Clinical pancreatitis | Permanently discontinue asparaginase use | [60–62] |
| | Hepatotoxicity, thrombohemorrhagic complications | Treatment delay may be required in subsequent chemotherapy | [60, 61, 63] |
| High-dose MTX | Acute kidney injury, high-grade myelosuppression, and severe mucositis | Withhold, reduce the dose, or delay subsequent chemotherapy | [64] |
| Combined 6-MP/low-dose MTX therapy | Moderate-to-severe hematological toxicities, infections, and non-infectious toxicities (e.g., oral ulcers, cholestatic jaundice) | Withhold, reduce the dose, or delay subsequent chemotherapy | [65] |
| Cytarabine | High-dose: myelotoxicity, gastrointestinal toxicity (e.g., oral mucositis, diarrhea, and intestinal injury), infections, and neurotoxicity | In severe cases: withhold, reduce the drug dose, or delay subsequent chemotherapy | [66] |
| | Standard-dose: myelosuppression and gastrointestinal toxicity | In severe cases: withhold, reduce the drug dose, or delay subsequent chemotherapy | [66] |
| | Low-dose: myelosuppression | In severe cases: withhold, reduce the drug dose, or delay subsequent chemotherapy | [66] |
| Thiopurines | Myelosuppression, hepatotoxicity, gastrointestinal toxicity, and hypoglycemia | In severe cases: withhold, reduce the dose, or add allopurinol | [67] |
| Azacitidine | Severe myelosuppression, high-grade gastrointestinal toxicity, and other adverse reactions | Interrupt treatment, reduce the dose or the treatment duration, or discontinue the drug | [33] |
| Anthracyclines | Myelosuppression, cardiotoxicity and gastrointestinal toxicity | Reducing the dose, controlling the infusion rate, using cardioprotective agents (e.g., iron chelator dexrazoxane), or substituting them with novel anthracycline analogues, liposomal preparations, or even non-anthracycline chemotherapeutic drugs | [68, 69] |
| Vinca alkaloids | Neurotoxicity, gastrointestinal distress, hepatotoxicity, hematological abnormalities, and cardiovascular toxicity | In cases with severe toxicities: discontinuing or delaying chemotherapy, adjusting the dose, using alternative therapy (e.g., replacement of vincristine with vindesine in patients with Charcot–Marie–Tooth disease), or substitution with specific dosage forms (e.g., liposomal vincristine) | [70] |

| Chemotherapy drug | Toxicity | Potential treatment modification associated with toxicity | Reference |
|---|---|---|---|
| Alkylating agents | Severe hematologic adverse events, infections, gastrointestinal intolerance, urinary tract toxicity, and neurologic adverse effects | Treatment suspension or dose reduction | [71] |
| Corticosteroids | Infections, psychological abnormalities, and bone toxicities | Dose reduction, treatment discontinuation, alternating daily schedules, or substitution of steroids (e.g., replacement of dexamethasone with prednisone) | [72] |
| Intrathecal chemotherapy | Chemical arachnoiditis, spinal cord lesions, seizures, and encephalopathy | Reducing the intrathecal (IT) drug dose or prolonging the intervals between IT chemotherapy cycles; dose adjustment of the systemically administered medications may also be considered | [95] |

*Abbreviations: MTX, methotrexate; 6-MP, 6-mercaptopurine.*

**Table 3.**
*Toxicity-induced treatment modifications for commonly used chemotherapeutic agents in leukemia.*

of asparaginase discontinuation on patient outcomes was evaluated in that study, and their results showed that discontinuation compromised EFS in T-ALL patients, which was in line with another study [5], but such an effect was not observed in those with T-lymphoblastic lymphoma [28].

Asparaginase-induced pancreatitis can be severe and life-threatening if not recognized and treated promptly. Usually, elevation in serum amylase and/or lipase alone, without clinical symptoms or imaging signs (i.e., chemical pancreatitis), does not necessitate asparaginase discontinuation [75]. However, for severe pancreatitis (i.e., clinical pancreatitis or symptomatic pancreatitis), permanent discontinuation is often required due to the high rate (approximately 50% or greater) of recurrence after re-exposure in subsequent chemotherapy cycles [60].

Patients treated with asparaginase may experience hypersensitivity reactions such as anaphylaxis, bronchospasm, angioedema, and urticaria, which often lead to modifications in treatment [77]. In addition to premedicating patients with anti-allergic agents such as antihistamines and corticosteroids before starting asparaginase, switching to a different preparation may be considered to alleviate clinical hypersensitivity reactions. There are three main formulations of asparaginase used in clinical applications. The pegylated form of *Escherichia coli* (*E. coli*)-derived asparaginase (pegaspargase) is a common choice of preparation due to its prolonged retention time and potentially reduced immunogenicity relative to native *E. coli* asparaginase. The asparaginase preparation derived from *Erwinia chrysanthemi* (*Erwinia* asparaginase), with only limited cross-reactivity, may be used as a substitute to reduce the subsequent risk of hypersensitivity reactions to native *E. coli* asparaginase or pegaspargase [78].

Hepatotoxicity and thrombohemorrhagic complications are the other two common AEs associated with asparaginase administration [79]. Both toxicities are usually thought to be dose-related. For severe acute hepatotoxicity (e.g., high-grade transaminitis, hyperbilirubinemia, or liver steatosis) or high-grade thrombotic and hemorrhagic complications, treatment delay may be required for subsequent chemotherapy. Considering asparaginase is a critical component of contemporary ALL regimens and unnecessary treatment modification may compromise the regimen's efficacy, dose reduction or discontinuation of asparaginase should be performed with caution [60, 61, 63]. The choice of intervention depends on the severity and resolution of toxicity, as well as the approach of the local protocol followed by the clinician.

### 3.2 Methotrexate

MTX, given intravenously in high doses (defined as a dose ≥500 mg/m$^2$), or orally (e.g., 20 mg/m$^2$) and intrathecally (e.g., 12 mg) in low doses, is an essential component of the intensive or maintenance treatment phase for ALL and lymphoma. MTX-associated toxicity carries the potential for treatment modifications, such as subsequent chemotherapy delays and dose reductions.

Patients receiving high-dose MTX (HD-MTX) therapy can experience serious toxicities such as acute kidney injury (AKI), high-grade myelosuppression, hepatotoxicity, and gastrointestinal toxicity, even with appropriate supportive care measures. MTX is eliminated primarily through the kidneys, so prolonged renal dysfunction leads to delayed clearance of MTX, which can further worsen or exacerbate its other toxicities. In patients with effusions, MTX is distributed in the effusion and leaks out continuously, exposing normal tissues to cumulative toxic amounts of the drug. Under these circumstances, aggressive management approaches (e.g., adequate hydration, urinary alkalinization to a urine pH >7, high-dose leucovorin rescue, timely glucarpidase administration, and/or hemodialysis) might be indicated [64]. Besides causing interruption or delaying cancer treatment, renal injury or MTX excretion delay can also lead to dose reduction or omission in subsequent chemotherapy, but treatment outcomes may be adversely affected [64]. Almost all patients treated with HD-MTX have some degree of acute elevations in serum transaminases or bilirubin, but these increments are usually transient, resolve spontaneously within one to two weeks, and do not lead to chronic liver disease. Therefore, it is unlikely that further intervention or dose adjustment in subsequent courses of HD-MTX will be needed. Accordingly, most study protocols do not recommend dose reduction or discontinuation in cases of high liver enzymes without evidence of severe hepatic dysfunction. Evident myelosuppression and mucositis can pose significant burdens for patients that may indicate the need for prompt interventions to reduce toxicity. In severe cases, suspending MTX infusion or delaying subsequent chemotherapy may be warranted, but these treatment modifications are largely empirical.

The combination of daily oral (e.g., 50 to 75 mg/m$^2$) 6-MP and weekly oral low-dose (20 to 40 mg/m$^2$) MTX, typically delivered for two to three years, is the mainstay in the maintenance treatment phase of ALL [80]. Although dose intensities in this phase are relatively lower, patients continue to experience a variety of side effects. Toxicities associated with this treatment modality include hematological toxicities (e.g., leukopenia, thrombocytopenia), hepatotoxicity, and mucositis [65]. During maintenance therapy, suitably lower white blood cell levels (e.g., between 1.5 and 3.0 (or 3.5) × $10^9$/L) and/or absolute neutrophil count (e.g., 0.75 to 1.5 × $10^9$/L) have been shown to be associated with a reduced risk of disease relapse [65, 80]. Accordingly, dose adjustments of 6-MP and MTX require individualization based on clinical status and blood count parameters (in particular, absolute neutrophil count), endeavoring to titrate and modify doses based on patients' tolerance [65]. For moderate-to-severe hematological toxicities, infections necessitating hospitalization, and clinically significant non-hematological toxicities (e.g., oral ulcers, cholestatic jaundice), doses of 6-MP and MTX may be reduced, or treatment may be delayed or withheld [65].

### 3.3 Thiopurines

The thiopurine antimetabolites 6-MP and 6-thioguanine (6-TG) have long been used for the treatment of acute leukemias. They are often prescribed as a component of regimens for the intensive and/or maintenance phase of treatment in patients with ALL and AML [67, 81]. Thiopurines are generally well tolerated, with myelotoxicity being the most common AE that potentially necessitates dose adjustment depending on the degree of myelosuppression. Non-hematological toxicities, such as hepatotoxicity, gastrointestinal toxicity (e.g., nausea, mucositis, and abdominal pain), and hypoglycemia, have also been associated with thiopurine treatment. Hepatotoxicity mainly manifests as mild elevations of serum aminotransferases without signs of severe hepatic dysfunction. In severe cases of such toxicities, discontinuation of therapy or dose reduction of the drugs may be required to allow recovery. For patients intolerant to 6-MP due to high 6-methylmercaptopurine (6-MMP) levels, the addition of allopurinol may also be considered [67, 82]. As the polymorphisms of the metabolizing enzymes (e.g., thiopurine methyltransferase (TPMT) and nudix hydrolase 15 (NUDT15)) and the levels of metabolites are implicated in the occurrence of certain thiopurine toxicities, genotype/phenotype status testing and TDM are often used to guide the dosing of these drugs [83].

### 3.4 Cytarabine

Different schedules and dose-intensities of Ara-C are widely used as a component of multi-agent chemotherapy regimens for the treatment of leukemias and lymphomas [84]. For instance, intermediate to high-dose (e.g., 2 to 6 g/($m^2$ day) for several cycles) Ara-C is frequently used in consolidation and salvage programs or as a remission induction component in relapsed or refractory acute leukemias, while low to standard-dose schemes (e.g., ≤200 mg/($m^2$ day) for consecutive days) are often adopted as essential components of induction schemes for AML patients.

The toxicity profile of Ara-C is contingent on the schedule and dose of administration [66]. When Ara-C is used at high doses, the potential side effects that may limit dosage and duration include severe myelotoxicity, gastrointestinal toxicity (e.g., oral mucositis, diarrhea, and intestinal injury), infections, and neurotoxicity [31]. Other adverse effects, such as ocular toxicity, skin rash, and elevation of hepatic enzymes, are also relatively frequent, but they usually do not lead to treatment modifications since the majority of them are reversible or can be prevented by prophylactic measures. With standard-dose regimens, the major serious toxicities of Ara-C are myelosuppression and gastrointestinal toxicity. Low-dose Ara-C is generally well tolerated, with the principal toxicity being myelosuppression. When these severe toxicities occur, withholding, reducing the drug dose, or delaying subsequent chemotherapy may be warranted.

### 3.5 Anthracyclines

Anthracyclines (e.g., daunorubicin, doxorubicin, idarubicin, or mitoxantrone) rank among the most effective and widely used anti-neoplastic agents in hematologic malignancies. They are often included in the regimens for remission induction or consolidation chemotherapy of ALL, AML, and APL. However, their clinical use is limited by a variety of toxic effects. Typical toxicities that often limit the maximum dose and the overall length of treatment include acute myelosuppression, cardiotoxicity, and gastrointestinal toxicities (e.g., oral ulcers, diarrhea) [68, 69]. Other adverse effects of this class of agents are liver injury and kidney damage, the majority of which are mild and reversible.

Despite the use of treatment measures such as hematopoietic colony-stimulating factors (CSFs) or platelet transfusions, recovery of blood cells in patients with myelosuppression can still take a longer time, potentially leading to delays in subsequent chemotherapy courses and/or reductions in relative dose intensity [85].

The development of cardiotoxicity from antineoplastic therapy is associated with certain important risk factors, such as higher cumulative dose, infusion schedule, and preexisting cardiac disorder [86]. In clinical practice, anthracyclines are usually not given in excess of the recommended maximum cumulative dose (e.g., doxorubicin 450 to 550 mg/m$^2$, epirubicin 900 to 1,000 mg/m$^2$) [69, 87]. In addition to limiting drug doses, other approaches, such as controlling the infusion rate, using cardioprotective agents (e.g., the iron chelator dexrazoxane), or substituting them with novel anthracycline analogues, liposomal preparations, or even non-anthracycline chemotherapeutic drugs (e.g., gemcitabine), may also serve as adjustment strategies for subsequent chemotherapy, although the benefits of these strategies are controversial in some settings [87, 88].

### 3.6 Vinca alkaloids

Vinca alkaloids (e.g., vincristine, vindesine, and vinblastine) are commonly used as part of multidrug combination regimens for the treatment of hematologic malignancies. However, vinca alkaloid therapies are associated with a variety of side effects that can affect treatment adherence or impair clinical benefit.

Neurotoxicities, specifically peripheral and autonomic neuropathy, are among the most common AEs associated with vinca alkaloid therapy. Higher doses of drugs, the presence of preexisting neuropathy, hepatic and renal dysfunction, genetic polymorphisms in drug-metabolizing enzymes (e.g., lower expression of CYP3A4 and CYP3A5), and the concomitant use of certain agents, such as azole antifungals, have been shown to increase the risk of neurotoxicity [70]. For example, to reduce the probability of developing acute neurotoxicity, a maximum single dose of 2 mg is recommended for vincristine [89]. Additionally, potential neuroprotectants such as glutamine, acetyl-L-carnitine, and vitamins B12 and B6 can also be applied to relieve vinca alkaloid-induced neuropathy, although more convincing clinical evidence is needed to confirm their effectiveness [89].

Apart from neurotoxicity, other acute toxicities, such as gastrointestinal distress, hepatotoxicity, bone marrow suppression, and cardiovascular effects, may also present during treatment with vinca alkaloid chemotherapeutic agents. In cases of severe toxicity effects, discontinuing or delaying chemotherapy, adjusting the dose, using alternative therapy (e.g., replacement of vincristine with vindesine in patients with Charcot-Marie-Tooth disease), or substitution with specific dosage forms (e.g., liposomal vincristine) may be considered to control the AEs.

### 3.7 Alkylating agents

Alkylating agents, in particular nitrogen mustards (e.g., cyclophosphamide, ifosfamide, bendamustine, chlorambucil, and melphalan), are among the most valuable cytotoxic drugs for the treatment of patients with hematologic malignancies, including multiple myeloma, lymphomas, and certain leukemias [90]. For example, alkylating agents, usually in combination with other agents such as corticosteroids, nucleoside analogues, or monoclonal antibodies (e.g., rituximab), are an essential component of standard therapy in B-cell CLL (B-CLL) [91]. However, the use of alkylating agents is constrained by several severe side effects. Acute toxicities that may warrant treatment modifications (e.g., treatment suspension, dose reduction) of these compounds include severe hematologic AEs (leukopenia or neutropenia, thrombocytopenia or anemia), infections, gastrointestinal intolerance (nausea, vomiting, and diarrhea), urinary tract toxicity (nephrotoxicity, hemorrhagic cystitis, dysuria, and hematuria), and neurologic adverse effects [71]. For example, in advanced CLL patients treated with bendamustine or chlorambucil, approximately one-third of patients required at least one dose reduction, primarily due to neutropenia and thrombocytopenia [92]. Treatment suspension or discontinuation may also be considered according to patient performance status and comorbidities, for instance, in the setting of severe AEs, including hematological and non-hematological toxicities [93, 94].

In addition to antineoplastic drug modifications that are commonly used during toxicity management, other preventive or treatment measures, such as the use of prophylactic hyperuricemic and anti-infective therapy, and the concurrent application of an acrolein metabolite-inactivating agent (e.g., mesna), granulocyte CSFs (G-CSFs), erythropoietin, and antiemetics, may also be considered for patients undergoing alkylator-based therapy.

### 3.8 Corticosteroids

In addition to being employed for anaphylaxis management and symptom control/prophylaxis of cancer or chemotherapy-related complications, including nausea and vomiting, cerebral edema, pain, and fatigue, corticosteroids are widely used as a part of the anticancer treatment in various hematologic malignancies, such as induction or maintenance therapy for acute leukemia. Common corticosteroids used for the treatment of hematologic malignancies include hydrocortisone, prednisone, dexamethasone, and methylprednisolone.

Numerous short- and long-term side effects may occur during corticosteroid therapy, such as infection, hypertension, hyperglycemia, hyperlipidemia, psychological abnormalities, and osteonecrosis [72]. The toxic effects of glucocorticoids vary based on patient characteristics (e.g., performance status, organ function), dose administered, treatment duration, and the specific combination chemotherapy regimen used [95]. For mild-to-moderate adverse reactions (e.g., hypertension, hyperglycemia, hyperlipidemia), the symptoms usually return to normal when treatment finishes. When severe AEs occur, clinical decisions are often adjusted based on the clinician's experience and local policies to be followed. Other than symptomatic treatment and supportive care, interventions to cope with these complications may also include treatment modification approaches, such as dose reduction, treatment cessation, alternating daily schedules, or substitution of steroids in the treatment program (e.g., replacement of dexamethasone with prednisone) [72]. In addition, prophylactic or concomitant treatment with antimicrobials (e.g., antibiotics and antifungal drugs) might be indicated in patients with high-risk or known infections undergoing corticosteroid therapy [96].

### 3.9 IT chemotherapy

The CNS is considered a unique sanctuary site for hematologic malignancies. Apart from intensive systemic chemotherapy, repeated IT chemotherapy has been an important approach for the prophylaxis and treatment of CNS involvement in patients with ALL or aggressive lymphoma [73]. Different IT chemotherapy regimens have been formulated, which may depend on the type of disease, patient characteristics, and whether they are used for prophylaxis or treatment. Traditionally, the drugs used for IT administration have been MTX, Ara-C, and glucocorticoids (e.g., hydrocortisone, prednisolone, dexamethasone, and methylprednisolone), often used in combination and administered based on age rather than body weight or body surface area, called Triple IT therapy (TIT) [97]. Other medications used for IT administration in hematologic malignancies include the controlled-release formulations of Ara-C (liposomal cytarabine), monoclonal antibodies (e.g., rituximab), and thiotepa [97, 98].

Although IT chemotherapy is generally safe, toxicities associated with it have also been observed, especially when administered in conjunction with other drugs that can cross the blood–brain barrier. Among adult patients receiving IT chemotherapy, at least one adverse reaction may occur after approximately one-third of IT treatment doses [99]. The most common and potentially serious effects of IT chemotherapy are headache, nausea, vomiting, and fever, which may be associated with chemical arachnoiditis [97, 99]. More severe neurological complications associated with IT administration have also been reported, such as spinal cord lesions, encephalopathy, convulsions, and long-term neurocognitive deficits [73, 97, 100].

Risk factors for the development of neurotoxicity related to IT treatment include the use of high doses, more frequent administrations, and CNS involvement [99, 101]. Therefore, the management of neurotoxicity mainly relies on reducing the IT drug dose or prolonging the intervals between IT chemotherapy cycles. In addition, as IT treatment is usually used in combination with high-dose intravenous therapy with good CNS penetration, dose adjustment of the systemically administered medications may also be considered.

## 4. Discussion

Hematologic malignancies pose a serious threat to human health. Due to constraints such as age, availability of suitable donors, socioeconomic status, treatment facilities, and other infrastructures, the majority of patients with hematologic malignancies still opt for non-transplant therapy. Multi-agent combination chemotherapy is widely used for the treatment of many hematologic malignancies (e.g., ALL, AML, NHL, and HL). For symptomatic or progressive CLL or CML, chemotherapy and alternative regimens, including molecular targeted therapy and immunotherapeutic approaches, may be recommended as strategies to improve survival.

Chemotherapy is a double-edged sword. While chemotherapeutic drugs are effective at killing tumor cells, they also inevitably cause damage to healthy tissues. Therefore, patients undergoing chemotherapy for hematologic malignancies often experience a variety of toxicities, the occurrence of which may be associated with multiple factors, including treatment regimens, timing of drug administration, patient-related factors (e.g., clinical status, comorbidities, and genetic polymorphisms affecting drug metabolism and clearance), as well as the quality of supportive care measures. The development of toxicities not only increases mortality rates but can also lead to dose reductions, treatment delays, premature discontinuation of therapy, or even substitution or omission of specific chemotherapy agents in subsequent treatment phases.

For the sake of safety, good patient performance status is usually required before starting each course or cycle of treatment (e.g., no severe infection, absolute neutrophil count $\geq 0.5 \times 10^9$/L or platelet count $\geq 100 \times 10^9$/L) [22]. Therefore, a mandatory rest period (e.g., two to four weeks) between chemotherapy cycles or treatment stages is necessary to allow normal tissues to recover from toxic events [10, 18, 102]. However, for a specific individual, the timing of initiating the next chemotherapy cycle depends on their overall health status and bone marrow recovery. Due to challenges in predicting treatment-related toxicities in advance, in most cases, when patients do not have serious complications before chemotherapy, drugs are often initially given at conventional dosages or intervals without modification.

Apart from conventional prognostic factors (e.g., adverse clinical and biological features, lack of access to effective treatment approaches, and inadequate supportive care), treatment-related morbidity events and consequent chemotherapy modifications are additional concerns that may influence outcomes in hematologic malignancies. However, potential biases may exist when evaluating treatment modifications, such as the definitions of dose reduction, treatment delay, and survival outcomes, which may contribute to the inconsistent findings regarding the impact of such adjustments on clinical outcomes [19, 29, 41].

The discrepancy in the impact of delay on outcomes may reflect differences in treatment intensity or drug exposure across studies. Most studies hold that treatment delay during intensive phases would cause inferior survival outcomes, potentially due to insufficient systemic exposure to therapeutic medications during the prolonged overall therapy duration caused by treatment interruptions. This suggests that, to maintain dose-intense chemotherapy, unnecessary treatment interruptions should be avoided, and protocol adherence should be ensured when mild toxicities occur. The seemingly paradoxical observation that children with longer treatment interruptions due to toxicity during the maintenance phase of ALL had better survival outcomes or fewer relapses [21, 29] implies that the intensity of maintenance chemotherapy may not have been sufficient for certain pediatric patients, possibly due to suboptimal chemotherapy exposure and reduced early toxicity. On the contrary, in the study conducted by Mangum et al. [27], who evaluated the impact of treatment delays on clinical outcomes, the authors found that prolonged delays before maintenance therapy did not affect survival, but extreme toxicities necessitating major therapy modifications were associated with significantly worse survival outcomes. However, it should be noted that most of the aforementioned studies are single-institutional and retrospective, with a relatively limited number of cases. Broader analyses involving larger patient cohorts and multi-center studies would be highly beneficial.

It should be noted that treatment modifications, such as schedule delays, drug substitutions, or dose omissions, can be caused not only by treatment-related toxicities (e.g., infections or organ damage) but also by non-medical reasons, such as financial difficulties, delayed insurance approval, lack of logistical support resources (e.g., drug shortages, bed unavailability, limited laboratory capacity, unavailable appointments), weekend admissions, and delays in the pre-chemotherapy phase (e.g., visit delays, diagnosis delays, treatment initiation delays) [103, 104]. Therefore, an important consideration in investigating treatment modifications during combination chemotherapy is identifying the drug causing toxicity and ruling out noncompliance. However, many studies failed to make a strict distinction between toxicity-induced delays and those caused by non-medical reasons when investigating the association of delays and clinical outcomes [5, 20]. Suarez et al. [26] pointed out that treatment delays, irrespective of their cause, are a major predictor of treatment failure.

As treatment modifications may signal poor patient performance status or intolerance to cytotoxic agents, and may also indicate suboptimal dose-intensive therapy, accurate risk stratification is often required to predict disease outcomes and guide treatment strategy selection. Individualizing chemotherapy regimens based on genetic characteristics and environmental factors to optimize dose intensity may help reduce the risk of severe complications and thus lower the likelihood of treatment modifications.

This review has several limitations. First, due to significant heterogeneity across studies in terms of treatment regimens, patient demographics, and outcome definitions, a formal meta-analysis was not conducted. Consequently, it was not possible to draw specific conclusions regarding the impact of treatment modification on clinical outcomes. Second, many of the included studies were conducted at single institutions and were retrospective in design, often with limited sample sizes. Although these studies offer valuable insights, they are susceptible to confounding factors and bias, which may limit the strength of the conclusions drawn. Third, the rapid progress in the treatment of hematologic malignancies means that some of the included studies may not reflect the most current clinical practices or technologies. Finally, the literature search was conducted and limited to PubMed and Google Scholar and restricted to the English language, which may have excluded relevant studies from other databases and publications in non-English languages, potentially introducing selection bias and limiting the reliability of the conclusions.

## 5. Conclusion

Although emerging treatment options such as targeted therapy, immunotherapy, CAR-T therapy, and stem cell transplantation are available, conventional combination chemotherapy remains crucial and widely used in leukemia management, particularly for acute leukemia subtypes. However, treatment modifications due to toxicities are common during chemotherapy. Considering the potential impact of treatment modification on clinical prognosis, further attention should be paid to this issue to achieve an optimal balance between efficacy and toxicity throughout the treatment course in the future.

## Author details

Dao-Hai Cheng[1*] and Wen-Ling Chen[2*†]

1 The First Affiliated Hospital of Guangxi Medical University, Department of Pharmacy, Nanning, China

2 Department of Postgraduate and Continuing Education after Graduation, The First Affiliated Hospital of Guangxi Medical University, Nanning, China

[†] Present address: Healthcare Management Section, Logistics and Infrastructure Department, Guangxi Medical University, Nanning, China

*Address all correspondence to: chengdaohai@gxmu.edu.cn, 489525685@qq.com

## References

[1] Tietsche de Moraes Hungria V, Chiattone C, Pavlovsky M, Abenoza LM, Agreda GP, Armenta J, Arrais C, Avendaño Flores O, Barroso F, Basquiera AL, Cao C, Cugliari MS, Enrico A, Foggliatto LM, Galvez KM, Gomez D, Gomez A, de Iracema D, Farias D, Lopez L, Mantilla WA, Martínez D, Mela MJ, Miguel CE, Ovilla R, Palmer L, Pavlovsky C, Ramos C, Remaggi G, Santucci R, Schusterschitz S, Sossa CL, Tuna-Aguilar E, Vela J, Santos T, de la Mora O, Machnicki G, Fernandez M, Barreyro P. Epidemiology of hematologic malignancies in real-world settings: Findings from the hemato-oncology latin america observational registry study. Journal of Global Oncology. 2019;**5**:1–19. DOI: 10.1200/JGO.19.00025

[2] Zhang N, Wu J, Wang Q, Liang Y, Li X, Chen G, Ma L, Liu X, Zhou F. Global burden of hematologic malignancies and evolution patterns over the past 30 years. Blood Cancer Journal. 2023;**13(1)**: 82. DOI: 10.1038/s41408-023-00853-3

[3] Bröckelmann PJ. Hodgkin lymphoma: Great progress with room for improvement. Nature Reviews Clinical Oncology. 2025;**22(6)**:379–381. DOI: 10.1038/s41571-025-01012-2

[4] Kantarjian H, Kadia T, DiNardo C, Daver N, Borthakur G, Jabbour E, Garcia-Manero G, Konopleva M, Ravandi F. Acute myeloid leukemia: Current progress and future directions. Blood Cancer Journal. 2021;**11(2)**: 41. DOI: 10.1038/s41408-021-00425-3

[5] Duffy C, Graetz DE, Lopez AMZ, Carrillo AK, Job G, Chen Y, Devidas M, Leon SA, Bonzi SA, Flores PC, Torres LE, Broncano EH, Jaramillo SJ, Zelada MO, Novoa RR, Samudio A, Sánchez-Fernandez G, Villanueva E, Metzger ML, Friedrich P, Jeha S. Retrospective analysis of outcomes for pediatric acute lymphoblastic leukemia in South American centers. Frontiers in Oncology. 2023;13:1254233. DOI: 10.3389/fonc.2023.1254233

[6] Malard F, Mohty M. Acute lymphoblastic leukaemia. The Lancet. 2020;**395**(10230):1146–1162. DOI: 10.1016/S0140-6736(19)33018-1

[7] Wenge DV, Wethmar K, Klar CA, Kolve H, Sauer T, Angenendt L, Evers G, Call S, Kerkhoff A, Khandanpour C, Kessler T, Mesters R, Schliemann C, Mikesch JH, Reicherts C, Brüggemann M, Berdel WE, Lenz G, Stelljes M. Characteristics and outcome of elderly patients (>55 Years) with acute lymphoblastic leukemia. Cancers (Basel). 2022;**14**(3):565. DOI: 10.3390/cancers14030565

[8] de Leeuw DC, Ossenkoppele GJ, Janssen JJWM. Older patients with acute myeloid leukemia deserve individualized treatment. Current Oncology Reports. 2022;**24**(11):1387–1400. DOI: 10.1007/s11912-022-01299-9

[9] Malczewska M, Kośmider K, Bednarz K, Ostapińska K, Lejman M, Zawitkowska J. Recent advances in treatment options for childhood acute lymphoblastic leukemia. Cancers (Basel). 2022;**14**(8):2021. DOI: 10.3390/cancers14082021

[10] Özdemir ZC, Kar YD, Turhan AB, Bör Ö. Assessment of hematological toxicity in children with acute lymphoblastic leukemia, receiving treatment with ALL IC-BFM 2009

protocol. Open Access Library Journal. 2017;**4**(8):e3807. DOI: 10.4236/oalib.1103807

[11] Ali AM, Adam H, Hailu D, Coenen MJH, Howe R, Abula T. Incidence and determinants of hematotoxicity in acute lymphoblastic leukemia children who received 6-mercaptopurine based maintenance therapy in Addis Ababa, Ethiopia. Plos One. 2023;**18**(6): e0286544. DOI: 10.1371/journal.pone.0286544

[12] Zawitkowska J, Lejman M, Zaucha-prażmo A, Drabko K, Płonowski M, Bulsa J, Romiszewski M, Mizia-Malarz A, Kołtan A, Derwich K, Karolczyk G, Ociepa T, Ćwiklińska M, Trelińska J, Owoc-Lempach J, Niedźwiecki M, Kiermasz A, Kowalczyk J. Grade 3 and 4 toxicity profiles during therapy of childhood acute lymphoblastic leukemia. In Vivo. 2019;33(4):1333–1339. DOI: 10.21873/invivo.11608

[13] Demidowicz E, Bartoszewicz N, Czyżewski K, Cisek J, Dąbrowska A, Dębski R, Dziedzic M, Ewertowska M, Grześki E, Jatczak-Gaca A, kołtan A, kołtan S, Krenska A, Łęcka M, Księżniakiewicz P, Marjański A, Pogorzała M, Richert-przygońska M, Tejza B, Urbańczyk A, Żołnowska H, Wysocki M, Styczyński J. Acute non-hematological toxicity of intensive chemotherapy of acute lymphoblastic leukemia in children. Acta Haematologica Polonica. 2020;**51** **(3)**:164–171. DOI: 10.2478/ahp-2020-0029

[14] Orgel E, Sposto R, Malvar J, Seibel NL, Ladas E, Gaynon PS, Freyer DR. Impact on survival and toxicity by duration of weight extremes during treatment for pediatric acute lymphoblastic leukemia: A report from the Children's Oncology Group. Journal of Clinical Oncology. 2014;**32(13)**:1331–1337. DOI: 10.1200/JCO.2013.52.6962

[15] O'Connor D, Bate J, Wade R, Clack R, Dhir S, Hough R, Vora A, Goulden N, Samarasinghe S. Infection-related mortality in children with acute lymphoblastic leukemia: An analysis of infectious deaths on UKALL2003. Blood. 2014;**124(7)**:1056–1061. DOI: 10.1182/blood-2014-03-560847

[16] Kuderer NM, Dale DC, Crawford J, Cosler LE, Lyman GH. Mortality, morbidity, and cost associated with febrile neutropenia in adult cancer patients. Cancer. 2006;**106**(10): 2258–2266. DOI: 10.1002/cncr.21847

[17] Rokkanen R, Aarnivala H, Pokka T, Niinimäki R. Chemotherapy-related toxicities follow a typical pattern in children treated for acute lymphoblastic leukaemia. Acta Paediatrica. 2024;**113** (5):1103–1111. DOI: 10.1111/apa.17092

[18] Kumar AJ, Gimotty PA, Gelfand JM, Buck G, Rowe JM, Goldstone AH, Fielding A, Marks DI, Litzow M, Paietta E, Lazarus HM, Tallman MS, Luger SM, Loren AW. Delays in postremission chemotherapy for Philadelphia chromosome negative acute lymphoblastic leukemia are associated with inferior outcomes in patients who undergo allogeneic transplant: An analysis from ECOG 2993/MRC UK ALLXII. American Journal of Hematology. 2016;**91** **(11)**:1107–1112. DOI: 10.1002/ajh.24497

[19] Agrawal V, Kayal S, Ganesan P, Dubashi B. Chemotherapy delays are associated with inferior outcome in acute lymphoblastic leukemia: A retrospective study from a tertiary cancer center in South India. Indian Journal of Medical and Paediatric

Oncology. 2021;**42(1)**:51–60. DOI: 10.1055/s-0041-1729513

[20] Puła A, Zdunek M, Michalczyk K, Cichosz M, Młynarski W. Chemotherapy delays in children with acute lymphoblastic leukemia might influence the outcome of treatment. Acta Haematologica Polonica. 2022;**53** (2):141–148. DOI: 10.5603/AHP.a2022.0007

[21] Yeoh A, Collins A, Fox K, Shields S, Ritchie P, Kirby M, Revesz T. Treatment delay and the risk of relapse in pediatric acute lymphoblastic leukemia. Pediatric Hematology and Oncology. 2017;**34 (1)**:38–42. DOI: 10.1080/08880018.2016.1276235

[22] Laughton SJ, Ashton LJ, Kwan E, Norris MD, Haber M, Marshall GM. Early responses to chemotherapy of normal and malignant hematologic cells are prognostic in children with acute lymphoblastic leukemia. Journal of Clinical Oncology. 2005;**23**(10): 2264–2271. DOI: 10.1200/JCO.2005.04.012

[23] Koka A, Saygin C, Uzunaslan D, Ozdemir N, Apak H, Celkan T. A 17-year experience with ALL-BFM protocol in acute lymphoblastic leukemia: Prognostic predictors and interruptions during protocol. Leukemia Research. 2014;**38**(6):699–705. DOI: 10.1016/j.leukres.2014.03.016

[24] Cao L, Gao J, Gao W, Liu H, Lu J, Wang Y, He HL, Xiao PF, Li J, Li JQ, Hu SY. Effect of chemotherapy course delay on the relapse of paediatric B-cell acute lymphoblastic leukemia. Zhongguo Shi, Yan Xue, Ye Xue, Za Zhi. 2022;**30(4)**:1034–1039. DOI: 10.19746/j.cnki.issn.1009-2137.2022.04.010

[25] Zhang QY, Lyu XY, Wang YZ, Li ZJ. Analysis of correlation between interval time of chemotherapy and prognosis in patients with acute leukemia. Zhongguo Shi Yan Xue Ye Xue Za Zhi. 2021;**29**(3):709–714. DOI: 10.19746/j.cnki.issn.1009-2137.2021.03.009

[26] Suarez A, Piña M, Nichols-Vinueza DX, Lopera J, Rengifo L, Mesa M, Cardenas M, Morrissey L, Veintemilla G, Vizcaino M, Del Toro L, Vicuna V, Fernandez J, Neuberg D, Stevenson K, Gutierrez A. A strategy to improve treatment-related mortality and abandonment of therapy for childhood ALL in a developing country reveals the impact of treatment delays. Pediatric Blood & Cancer. 2015;**62 (8)**:1395–1402. DOI: 10.1002/pbc.25510

[27] Mangum R, Chambers TM, Stevens A, Lynch RC, Burrows E, Miller TP, Getz KD, Aplenc R, Lupo PJ, Gramatges MMJ, Scheurer ME, Rabin KR. Delays in therapy do not impact survival in childhood acute lymphoblastic leukemia: A report from the learn consortium. Blood. 2019;**134 (Suppl 1)**:1304–1304. DOI: 10.1182/blood-2019-130351

[28] Ishida H, Imamura T, Kobayashi R, Hashii Y, Deguchi T, Miyamura T, Oda M, Yamamoto M, Okada K, Sano H, Koh K, Yuza Y, Watanabe K, Nishimura N, Takimoto T, Moriya-Saito A, Sekimizu M, Suenobu S, Sunami S, Horibe K. Differential impact of asparaginase discontinuation on outcomes of children with T-cell acute lymphoblastic leukemia and T-cell lymphoblastic lymphoma. Cancer Medicine. 2024;**13(12)**:e7246. DOI: 10.1002/cam4.7246

[29] de Oliveira BM, Valadares MTM, Silva MR, Viana MB. Compliance with a protocol for acute lymphoblastic

leukemia in childhood. Revista Brasileira de Hematologia E Hemoterapia. 2011;**33**(3):185–189. DOI: 10.5581/1516-8484.20110051

[30] Raychaudhuri S, Othus M, Percival M-EM, Garcia-Manero G, Appelbaum FR, Erba HP, Appelbaum J. Treatment discontinuation due to toxicity for patients with acute myeloid leukemia (AML) treated on SWOG S1203. Journal of Clinical Oncology. 2024;**42(Suppl 16)**:6529. DOI: 10.1200/JCO.2024.42.16_suppl.6529

[31] Lopes LM, Nucci M, Portugal RD. Toxicity and outcome of adults with acute myeloid leukemia receiving consolidation with high-dose cytarabine. Hematology, Transfusion and Cell Therapy. 2024;**46(4)**:397–401. DOI: 10.1016/j.htct.2023.07.007

[32] Sperr WR, Herndlhofer S, Gleixner K, Girschikofsky M, Weltermann A, Machherndl-Spandl S, Sliwa T, Poehnl R, Buxhofer-Ausch V, Strecker K, Hoermann G, Knoebl P, Jaeger U, Geissler K, Kundi M, Valent P. Intensive consolidation with G-CSF support: Tolerability, safety, reduced hospitalization, and efficacy in acute myeloid leukemia patients ≥60 years. American Journal of Hematology. 2017;**92(10)**:E567–E574. DOI: 10.1002/ajh.24847

[33] Ravandi F, Roboz GJ, Wei AH, Dehner H, Pocock C, Selleslag D, Montesinos P, Sayar H, Musso M, Figuera-Alvarez A, Safah H, Tse W, Sohn SK, Hiwase D, Chevassut T, Pierdomenico F, La Torre I, Skikne B, Bailey R, Zhong J, Beach CL, Dombret H. Management of adverse events in patients with acute myeloid leukemia in remission receiving oral azacitidine: Experience from the phase 3 randomized QUAZAR AML-001 trial. Journal of Hematology & Oncology. 2021;**14(1)**:133. DOI: 10.1186/s13045-021-01142-x

[34] Hillmen P, Pitchford A, Bloor A, Broom A, Young M, Kennedy B, Walewska R, Furtado M, Preston G, Neilson JR, Pemberton N, Sidra G, Morley N, Cwynarski K, Schuh A, Forconi F, Elmusharaf N, Paneesha S, Fox CP, Howard DR, Hockaday A, Brown JM, Cairns DA, Jackson S, Greatorex N, Webster N, Shingles J, Dalal S, Patten PEM, Allsup D, Rawstron A, Munir T. Ibrutinib and rituximab versus fludarabine, cyclophosphamide, and rituximab for patients with previously untreated chronic lymphocytic leukaemia (FLAIR): Interim analysis of a multicentre, open-label, randomised, phase 3 trial. The Lancet Oncology. 2023;**24(5)**:535–552. DOI: 10.1016/S1470-2045(23)00144-4

[35] Oliveira AC, Roncero JM, Ferra C, Do Nascimento J, Rodriguez-Luaces M, Encuentra M, Domingo-Domenech E, Lopez P, Gallardo D, Ribera JM, Sarrá J, Sureda A, González-Barca E. Front-line fludarabine-cyclophosphamide-rituximab (FCR) in 110 patients with chronic lymphocytic leukaemia (CLL): Real-life experience with long-term outcomes, toxicities and responses to second-line therapies. International Journal of Hematology. 2023;**117(3)**:388–397. DOI: 10.1007/s12185-022-03488-5

[36] Abaza Y, Kantarjian H, Alwash Y, Borthakur G, Champlin R, Kadia T, Garcia-Manero G, Daver N, Ravandi F, Verstovsek S, Burger J, Estrov Z, Ohanian M, Lim M, Pemmaraju N, Jabbour E, Cortes J. Phase I/II study of dasatinib in combination with decitabine in patients with accelerated or blast phase chronic myeloid leukemia. American Journal of

Hematology. 2020;**95(11)**:1288–1295. DOI: 10.1002/ajh.25939

[37] Oki Y, Kantarjian HM, Gharibyan V, Jones D, O'brien S, Verstovsek S, Cortes J, Morris GM, Garcia-Manero G, Issa JP. Phase II study of low-dose decitabine in combination with imatinib mesylate in patients with accelerated or myeloid blastic phase of chronic myelogenous leukemia. Cancer. 2007;**109(5)**:899–906. DOI: 10.1002/cncr.22470

[38] Strati P, Kantarjian H, Thomas D, O'brien S, Konoplev S, Jorgensen JL, Luthra R, Abruzzo L, Jabbour E, Quintas-Cardama A, Borthakur G, Faderl S, Ravandi F, Cortes J. HCVAD plus imatinib or dasatinib in lymphoid blastic phase chronic myeloid leukemia. Cancer. 2014;**120(3)**:373–380. DOI: 10.1002/cncr.28433

[39] Namjoshi NS, Keegan THM, Li QC, Chung JH, Rosenthal JL, Winestone LE, Muffly L, Malogolowkin MH, Alvarez EM. Treatment-related toxicities associated with hospitalization in children, adolescents, and young adults with acute lymphoblastic leukemia: Population level analysis. Leukemia & Lymphoma. 2022;**63(13)**:3191–3199. DOI: 10.1080/10428194.2022.2113533

[40] PDQ Pediatric Treatment Editorial Board. Childhood acute lymphoblastic leukemia treatment (PDQ®): Health professional version. In: PDQ Cancer Information Summaries. Bethesda (MD): National Cancer Institute (US). 2025. PMID: 26389206

[41] Toft N, Birgens H, Abrahamsson J, Griskevicius L, Hallböök H, Heyman M, Klausen TW, Johnsson G, Palk K, Pruunsild K, Quist-Paulsen P, Vaitkeviciene G, Vettenranta K, Asberg A, Helt LR, Frandsen T, Schmiegelow K. Toxicity profile and treatment delays in NOPHO ALL2008—comparing adults and children with Philadelphia chromosome-negative acute lymphoblastic leukemia. European Journal of Haematology. 2016;**96(2)**:160–169. DOI: 10.1111/ejh.12562

[42] Hashmi SK, Bodea J, Patni T, Angel S, Bhakta NH, Jeha S, Karol SE, Ribeiro RC, Rubnitz JE, Wolf J, Li Y, Pui CH, Hijano DR, Inaba H. COVID-19 in pediatric patients with acute lymphoblastic leukemia or lymphoma. JAMA Network Open. 2024;**7**(2):e2355727. DOI: 10.1001/jamanetworkopen.2023.55727

[43] Omar AA, Basiouny L, Elnoby AS, Zaki A, Abouzid M. St. Jude Total Therapy studies from I to XVII for childhood acute lymphoblastic leukemia: A brief review. Journal of the Egyptian National Cancer Institute. 2022;**34**(1):25. DOI: 10.1186/s43046-022-00126-3

[44] Derman BA, Streck M, Wynne J, Christ TN, Curran E, Stock W, Knoebel RW. Efficacy and toxicity of reduced vs. standard dose pegylated asparaginase in adults with Philadelphia chromosome-negative acute lymphoblastic leukemia. Leukemia & Lymphoma. 2020;**61(3)**:614–622. DOI: 10.1080/10428194.2019.1680839

[45] Tomizawa D. Evolution and optimization of therapies for acute lymphoblastic leukemia in infants. International Journal of Hematology. 2023;**117**(2):162–172. DOI: 10.1007/s12185-022-03502-w

[46] Salzer WL, Jones TL, Devidas M, Dreyer ZE, Gore L, Winick NJ, Sung L, Raetz E, Loh ML, Wang CY, De Lorenzo P, Valsecchi MG, Pieters R, Carroll WL, Hunger SP, Hilden JM, Brown P.

Decreased induction morbidity and mortality following modification to induction therapy in infants with acute lymphoblastic leukemia enrolled on AALL0631: A report from the Children's Oncology Group. Pediatric Blood & Cancer. 2015;**62(3)**:414–418. DOI: 10.1002/pbc.25311

[47] Shimony S, Stahl M, Stone RM. Acute myeloid leukemia: 2023 update on diagnosis, risk-stratification, and management. American Journal of Hematology. 2023;**98**(3):502–526. DOI: 10.1002/ajh.26822

[48] Jimenez-Chillon C, Dillon R, Russell N. Optimal post-remission consolidation therapy in patients with AML. Acta Haematologica. 2024;**147**(2):147–158. DOI: 10.1159/000535457

[49] PDQ Adult Treatment Editorial Board. Acute myeloid leukemia treatment (PDQ®): Health professional version. In: PDQ Cancer Information Summaries. Bethesda (MD): National Cancer Institute (US). 2025. PMID: 26389432

[50] Shadman M. Diagnosis and treatment of chronic lymphocytic leukemia: A review. Jama. 2023;**329**(11):918–932. DOI: 10.1001/jama.2023.1946

[51] PDQ Adult Treatment Editorial Board. Chronic lymphocytic leukemia treatment (PDQ®): Health professional version. In: PDQ Cancer Information Summaries. Bethesda (MD): National Cancer Institute (US). 2025. PMID: 26389470

[52] Keating MJ, OBrien S, Albitar M, Lerner S, Plunkett W, Giles F, Andreeff M, Cortes J, Faderl S, Thomas D, Koller C, Wierda W, Detry MA, Lynn A, Kantarjian H. Early results of a chemoimmunotherapy regimen of fludarabine, cyclophosphamide, and rituximab as initial therapy for chronic lymphocytic leukemia. Journal of Clinical Oncology. 2005;**23(18)**:4079–4088. DOI: 10.1200/JCO.2005.12.051

[53] Jabbour E, Kantarjian H. Chronic myeloid leukemia: 2025 update on diagnosis, therapy, and monitoring. American Journal of Hematology. 2024;**99**(11):2191–2212. DOI: 10.1002/ajh.27443

[54] Pamuk GE, Ehrlich LA. An overview of myeloid blast-phase chronic myeloid leukemia. Cancers (Basel). 2024;**16**(21):3615. DOI: 10.3390/cancers16213615

[55] Sembill S, Ampatzidou M, Chaudhury S, Dworzak M, Kalwak K, Karow A, Kiani A, Krumbholz M, Luesink M, Naumann-Bartsch N, De Moerloose B, Osborn M, Schultz KR, Sedlacek P, Giona F, Zwaan CM, Shimada H, Versluijs B, Millot F, Hijiya N, Suttorp M, Metzler M. Management of children and adolescents with chronic myeloid leukemia in blast phase: International pediatric CML expert panel recommendations. Leukemia. 2023;**37(3)**:505–517. DOI: 10.1038/s41375-023-01822-2

[56] Gyurkocza B, Sandmaier BM. Conditioning regimens for hematopoietic cell transplantation: One size does not fit all. Blood. 2014;**124**(3):344–353. DOI: 10.1182/blood-2014-02-514778

[57] Lee BJ, Griffin SP, Doh J, Ciurea SO, Jeyakumar D, Kongtim P, Naqvi K. Intensification of upfront chemotherapy for patients with myeloid blast phase CML: A single center

experience. Annals of Hematology. 2024;**103(12)**:5395–5403. DOI: 10.1007/s00277-024-06045-8

[58] Gagelmann N, Kröger N. Dose intensity for conditioning in allogeneic hematopoietic cell transplantation: Can we recommend "when and for whom" in 2021? Haematologica. 2021;**106** (7):1794–1804. DOI: 10.3324/haematol.2020.268839

[59] Bacher U, Klyuchnikov E, Wiedemann B, Kroeger N, Zander AR. Safety of conditioning agents for allogeneic haematopoietic transplantation. Expert Opinion on Drug Safety. 2009;**8**(3):305–315. DOI: 10.1517/14740330902918273

[60] Burke PW, Hoelzer D, Park JH, Schmiegelow K, Douer D. Managing toxicities with asparaginase-based therapies in adult ALL: Summary of an ESMO Open–Cancer Horizons roundtable discussion. ESMO Open. 2020;**5**(5): e000858. DOI: 10.1136/esmoopen-2020-000858

[61] Stock W, Douer D, De Angelo DJ, Arellano M, Advani A, Damon L, Kovacsovics T, Litzow M, Rytting M, Borthakur G, Bleyer A. Prevention and management of asparaginase/pegasparaginase-associated toxicities in adults and older adolescents: Recommendations of an expert panel. Leukemia & Lymphoma. 2011;**52** **(12)**:2237–2253. DOI: 10.3109/10428194.2011.596963

[62] Douer D, Gökbuget N, Stock W, Boissel N. Optimizing use of L-asparaginase–based treatment of adults with acute lymphoblastic leukemia. Blood Reviews. 2022;53:100908. DOI: 10.1016/j.blre.2021.100908

[63] Aldoss I, Douer D. How I treat the toxicities of pegasparaginase in adults with acute lymphoblastic leukemia. Blood. 2020;**135**(13):987–995. DOI: 10.1182/blood.2019002477

[64] Howard SC, McCormick J, Pui CH, Buddington RK, Harvey RD. Preventing and managing toxicities of high-dose methotrexate. The Oncologist. 2016;**21** (12):1471–1482. DOI: 10.1634/theoncologist.2015-0164

[65] Krishnan S, Mahadevan A, Mungle T, Gogoi MP, Saha V. Maintenance treatment in acute lymphoblastic leukemia: A clinical primer. Indian Journal of Pediatrics. 2024;**91**(1):47–58. DOI: 10.1007/s12098-023-04687-6

[66] Stentoft J. The toxicity of cytarabine. Drug Safety. 1990;**5**(1):7–27. DOI: 10.2165/00002018-199005010-00003

[67] Toksvang LN, Lee SHR, Yang JJ, Schmiegelow K. Maintenance therapy for acute lymphoblastic leukemia: Basic science and clinical translations. Leukemia. 2022;**36**(7):1749–1758. DOI: 10.1038/s41375-022-01591-4

[68] Hortobágyi GN. Anthracyclines in the treatment of cancer: An overview. Drugs. 1997;**54**(Suppl 4):1–7. DOI: 10.2165/00003495-199700544-00003

[69] Bayles CE, Hale DE, Konieczny A, Anderson VD, Richardson CR, Brown KV, Nguyen JT, Hecht J, Schwartz N, Kharel MK, Amissah F, Dowling TC, Nybo SE. Upcycling the anthracyclines: New mechanisms of action, toxicology, and pharmacology. Toxicology and Applied Pharmacology . 2023;459:116362. DOI: 10.1016/j.taap.2022.116362

[70] Chen RJ, Arora RD, Menezes RG. Vinca alkaloid toxicity. In: StatPearls. Treasure Island (FL): StatPearls Publishing. 2025. PMID: 32491774

[71] Karati D, Mahadik KR, Trivedi P, Kumar D. Alkylating agents, the road less traversed, changing anticancer therapy. Anti-Cancer Agents in Medicinal Chemistry. 2022;**22**(8): 1478–1495. DOI: 10.2174/1871520621666210811105344

[72] Rossi SJ, Schroeder TJ, Hariharan S, First MR. Prevention and management of the adverse effects associated with immunosuppressive therapy. Drug Safety. 1993;**9**(2):104–131. DOI: 10.2165/00002018-199309020-00004

[73] Kwong Y-L, Yeung DYM, Chan JCW. Intrathecal chemotherapy for hematologic malignancies: Drugs and toxicities. Annals of Hematology. 2009;**88**(3):193–201. DOI: 10.1007/s00277-008-0645-y

[74] Hijiya N, van der Sluis IM. Asparaginase-associated toxicity in children with acute lymphoblastic leukemia. Leukemia & Lymphoma. 2016;**57**(4):748–757. DOI: 10.3109/10428194.2015.1101098

[75] Pourhassan H, Douer D, Pullarkat V, Aldoss I. Asparaginase: How to better manage toxicities in adults. Current Oncology Reports. 2023;**25**(1):51–61. DOI: 10.1007/s11912-022-01345-6

[76] Elgehiny A, Hsu A, McCall D, Gibson A, Cuglievan B, Nunez C, Garcia MB, Castellanos L, Funck A, Razvi S. Severe hypertriglyceridemia secondary to long-acting asparaginase in pediatric patients with acute lymphoblastic leukemia. Journal of Pediatric Hematology/Oncology. 2025;**47(6)**: e215–e221. DOI: 10.1097/MPH.0000000000003077

[77] Heo Y-A, Syed YY, Keam SJ. Pegaspargase: A review in acute lymphoblastic leukaemia. Drugs. 2019;**79**(7):767–777. DOI: 10.1007/s40265-019-01120-1

[78] Pui CH, Liu Y, Relling MV. How to solve the problem of hypersensitivity to asparaginase? Pediatric Blood & Cancer. 2018;**65**(3):e26884. DOI: 10.1002/pbc.26884

[79] Bade NA, Lu C, Patzke CL, Baer MR, Duong VH, Law JY, Lee ST, Sausville EA, Zimrin AB, Duffy AP, Lawson J, Emadi A. Optimizing pegylated asparaginase use: An institutional guideline for dosing, monitoring, and management. Journal of Oncology Pharmacy Practice. 2020;**26(1)**:74–92. DOI: 10.1177/1078155219838316

[80] Schmiegelow K, Nielsen SN, Frandsen TL, Nersting J. Mercaptopurine/Methotrexate maintenance therapy of childhood acute lymphoblastic leukemia: Clinical facts and fiction. Journal of Pediatric Hematology/Oncology. 2014;**36**(7):503–517. DOI: 10.1097/MPH.0000000000000206

[81] Fotoohi AK, Coulthard SA, Albertioni F. Thiopurines: Factors influencing toxicity and response. Biochemical Pharmacology. 2010;**79**(9):1211–1220. DOI: 10.1016/j.bcp.2010.01.006

[82] Kamojjala R, Bostrom B. Allopurinol to prevent mercaptopurine adverse effects in children and young adults with acute lymphoblastic leukemia. Journal of Pediatric Hematology/Oncology. 2021;**43**(3):

95–100. DOI: 10.1097/MPH.0000000000002117

[83] Relling MV, Schwab M, Whirl-Carrillo M, Suarez-Kurtz G, Pui CH, Stein CM, Moyer AM, Evans WE, Klein TE, Antillon-Klussmann FG, Caudle KE, Kato M, Yeoh AEJ, Schmiegelow K, Yang JJ. Clinical pharmacogenetics implementation consortium guideline for thiopurine dosing based on TPMT and NUDT15 Genotypes: 2018 update. Clinical Pharmacology & Therapeutics. 2019;**105(5)**:1095–1105. DOI: 10.1002/cpt.1304

[84] Di Francia R, Crisci S, De Monaco A, Cafiero C, Re A, Iaccarino G, De Filippi R, Frigeri F, Corazzelli G, Micera A, Pinto A. Response and toxicity to cytarabine therapy in leukemia and lymphoma: From dose puzzle to pharmacogenomic biomarkers. Cancers (Basel). 2021;**13**(5):966. DOI: 10.3390/cancers13050966

[85] Sasse EC, Sasse AD, Brandalise S, Clark OA, Richards S. Colony stimulating factors for prevention of myelosupressive therapy induced febrile neutropenia in children with acute lymphoblastic leukaemia. Cochrane Database of Systematic Reviews. 2005;(3):CD004139. DOI: 10.1002/14651858.CD004139.pub2

[86] Chanan-Khan A, Srinivasan S, Czuczman MS. Prevention and management of cardiotoxicity from antineoplastic therapy. The Journal of Supportive Oncology. 2004;**2**(3):251–256; discussion 259-261, 264-266. PMID: 15328825

[87] Barry E, Alvarez JA, Scully RE, Miller TL, Lipshultz SE. Anthracycline-induced cardiotoxicity: Course, pathophysiology, prevention and management. Expert Opinion on Pharmacotherapy. 2007;**8**(8):1039–1058. DOI: 10.1517/14656566.8.8.1039

[88] Kesavan M, Eyre TA, Collins GP. Front-Line treatment of high grade B cell non-hodgkin lymphoma. Current Hematologic Malignancy Reports. 2019;**14**(4):207–218. DOI: 10.1007/s11899-019-00518-8

[89] Madsen ML, Due H, Ejskjær N, Jensen P, Madsen J, Dybkær K. Aspects of vincristine-induced neuropathy in hematologic malignancies: A systematic review. Cancer Chemotherapy and Pharmacology. 2019;**84**(3):471–485. DOI: 10.1007/s00280-019-03884-5

[90] Lehmann F, Wennerberg J. Evolution of nitrogen-based alkylating anticancer agents. Processes. 2021;**9**(2):377. DOI: 10.3390/pr9020377

[91] Kay NE. Purine analogue-based chemotherapy regimens for patients with previously untreated B-Chronic lymphocytic leukemia. Seminars in Hematology. 2006;**43(2 Suppl 2)**:S50–S54. DOI: 10.1053/j.seminhematol.2005.12.011

[92] Knauf WU, Lissichkov T, Aldaoud A, Liberati A, Loscertales J, Herbrecht R, Juliusson G, Postner G, Gercheva L, Goranov S, Becker M, Fricke HJ, Huguet F, Del Giudice I, Klein P, Tremmel L, Merkle K, Montillo M. Phase III randomized study of bendamustine compared with chlorambucil in previously untreated patients with chronic lymphocytic leukemia. Journal of Clinical Oncology. 2009;**27(26)**:4378–4384. DOI: 10.1200/JCO.2008.20.8389

[93] Hoy SM. Bendamustine: A review of its use in the management of chronic lymphocytic leukaemia, rituximab-refractory indolent non-

Hodgkin's lymphoma and multiple myeloma. Drugs. 2012;**72**(14): 1929–1950. DOI: 10.2165/11209510-000000000-00000

[94] Cheson BD, Brugger W, Damaj G, Dreyling M, Kahl B, Kimby E, Ogura M, Weidmann E, Wendtner CM, Zinzani PL. Optimal use of bendamustine in hematologic disorders: Treatment recommendations from an international consensus panel – An update. Leukemia & Lymphoma. 2016;**57(4)**:766–782. DOI: 10.3109/10428194.2015.1099647

[95] Inaba H, Pui C-H. Glucocorticoid use in acute lymphoblastic leukaemia. The Lancet Oncology. 2010;**11**(11):1096–1106. DOI: 10.1016/S1470-2045(10)70114-5

[96] Faggiano A, Mazzilli R, Natalicchio A, Adinolfi V, Argentiero A, Danesi R,D'Oronzo S, Fogli S, Gallo M, Giuffrida D, Gori S, Montagnani M, Ragni A, Renzelli V, Russo A, Silvestris N, Franchina T, Tuveri E, Cinieri S, Colao A, Giorgino FZatelli MC. Corticosteroids in oncology: Use, overuse, indications, contraindications. An Italian Association of Medical Oncology (AIOM)/ Italian Association of Medical Diabetologists (AMD)/ Italian Society of Endocrinology (SIE)/ Italian Society of Pharmacology (SIF) multidisciplinary consensus position paper. *Critical Reviews in Oncology/Hematology*. 2022;180:103826. DOI: 10.1016/j.critrevonc.2022.103826

[97] Olmos-Jiménez R, Espuny-Miró A, Cárceles Rodríguez C, Díaz-Carrasco MS. Practical aspects of the use of intrathecal chemotherapy. Farmacia Hospitalaria : Organo Oficial de Expresion Cientifica de la Sociedad Espanola de Farmacia Hospitalaria. 2017;**41**(1):105–129. DOI: 10.7399/fh.2017.41.1.10616

[98] Jamison T, Haque E, Muhsen IN, Samarkandi H, Fakih RE, Aljurf M. Revisiting intrathecal thiotepa: Efficacy and safety in secondary CNS malignancies. Medical Oncology. 2024;**41**(7):177. DOI: 10.1007/s12032-024-02401-w

[99] Byrnes DM, Vargas F, Dermarkarian C, Kahn R, Kwon D, Hurley J, Schatz JH. Complications of intrathecal chemotherapy in adults: Single-Institution experience in 109 consecutive patients. Journal of Oncology. 2019;**2019**:4047617. DOI: 10.1155/2019/4047617

[100] Thastrup M, Duguid A, Mirian C, Schmiegelow K, Halsey C. Central nervous system involvement in childhood acute lymphoblastic leukemia: Challenges and solutions. Leukemia. 2022;**36**(12):2751–2768. DOI: 10.1038/s41375-022-01714-x

[101] Verstappen CC, Heimans JJ, Hoekman K, Postma TJ. Neurotoxic complications of chemotherapy in patients with cancer: Clinical signs and optimal management. Drugs. 2003;**63**(15):1549–1563. DOI: 10.2165/00003495-200363150-00003

[102] Cunningham D, Hawkes EA, Jack A, Qian W, Smith P, Mouncey P, Pocock C, Ardeshna KM, Radford JA, McMillan A, Davies J, Turner D, Kruger A, Johnson P, Gambell J, Linch D. Rituximab plus cyclophosphamide, doxorubicin, vincristine, and prednisolone in patients with newly diagnosed diffuse large B-cell non-Hodgkin lymphoma: A phase 3 comparison of dose intensification

with 14-day versus 21-day cycles. The Lancet. 2013;**381(9880)**:1817–1826. DOI: 10.1016/S0140-6736(13)60313-X

[103] Abel GA, Friese CR, Magazu LS, Richardson LC, Fernandez ME, De Zengotita JJ, Earle CC. Delays in referral and diagnosis for chronic hematologic malignancies: A literature review. Leukemia & Lymphoma. 2008;**49** (7):1352–1359. DOI: 10.1080/10428190802124281

[104] Wahl SK, Gildengorin G, Feusner J. Weekend delay in initiation of chemotherapy for acute lymphoblastic leukemia: Does it matter? Journal of Pediatric Hematology/Oncology. 2012;**34**(1):e8–e11. DOI: 10.1097/MPH.0b013e31822e9c0b